THE AUTISTS

THE
AUTISTS

WOMEN ON THE SPECTRUM

Clara Törnvall

translated by Alice E. Olsson

SCRIBE

Melbourne • London

Scribe Publications
2 John St, Clerkenwell, London, WC1N 2ES, United Kingdom
18–20 Edward St, Brunswick, Victoria 3056, Australia
3754 Pleasant Ave, Suite 100, Minneapolis, Minnesota 55409, USA

First published in Swedish as *Autisterna: om kvinnor på spektrat* by Natur & Kultur 2021
Published by arrangement with Nordin Agency AB, Sweden

First published in English by Scribe 2023

Typeset in Garamond Premier Pro by the publishers

Printed and bound in the UK by CPI Group (UK) Ltd, Croydon CR0 4YY

Scribe is committed to the sustainable use of natural resources and the use of paper products
made responsibly from those resources.

978 1 914484 81 0 (UK edition)
978 1 957363 53 0 (US edition)
978 1 922585 89 9 (Australian edition)
978 1 761385 12 4 (ebook)

Catalogue records for this book are available from the National Library of Australia and the
British Library.

The cost of this translation was supported by a subsidy from the Swedish Arts Council,
gratefully acknowledged.

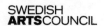

SWEDISH
ARTSCOUNCIL

scribepublications.co.uk
scribepublications.com
scribepublications.com.au

To Harry and Lydia

CONTENTS

INTRODUCTION

There ought, I thought, to be a ritual for being born twice
— patched, retreaded, and approved for the road.

SYLVIA PLATH, *THE BELL JAR*

'Let's go to page seven,' says the psychologist.

I browse among the pages on my lap. There it is, at the bottom: 'Autism, without accompanying intellectual impairment and without accompanying language impairment, level 1.'

'There's nothing else interfering,' the psychologist says kindly. 'No suspicions about other diagnoses.'

I read that I fulfil all seven diagnostic criteria for what used to be known as Asperger's syndrome. By a long shot, it seems. On one of the rating scales where a score of more than 77 points supports a diagnosis, I come in at 154. I feel like I've done well by being such a clear-cut case.

The assessment, which we are going through together, also includes a summary of my psychiatric history. It's aimed at others within the psychiatric services whom I may come into contact with in the future, the psychologist explains.

That won't happen, I think to myself. I will never again be in contact with the psychiatric services. This is it.

My past unfolds. It's like watching a film with an unexpected twist at the end. A revelation that overturns everything I thought I knew about the main characters and the plot. The hints foreshadowing the solution to the mystery suddenly appear in stark focus. They line up, one after another throughout the years. The signs have been there all along.

I have always known that I'm autistic. And yet I haven't had a clue.

Three months earlier, I walk through downtown Hagsätra, a suburb south of Stockholm. I step in under a roof, passing the supermarket and the pastry shop, my mind churning with the same three words: *This is it.* It happens sometimes — a sentence gets stuck in my head, a short loop repeating itself like an incantation.

The neuropsychiatric clinic is hard to find, despite the GPS in my phone. I spin a lap in the wrong direction through the downtown area and come to a stop, disoriented, in front of a statue titled *Girl with a Ball.* The girl is leaning forward, frozen, with her mouth shaped into an O. The fountain in front of her has been drained of water; the stream she blows is invisible.

I'm 42 years old and so tired of myself that I have just about had it. As far back as I can remember, I have suffered from anxiety: a sinkhole in the pit of my stomach that I'm so used to, it has become my ground state. The anxiety has nothing to do with my thoughts; it lives in me like an organism of its own. I'm not compulsive or hypochondriacal, not plagued by worry. I don't meditate on future disaster scenarios. But as I move through the world, I'm always uncertain. Every step I take is tentative, as though I'm walking on thin ice.

I'm constantly on edge and weighed down by a sorrow I don't understand. I sleep with my fists clenched at night. For periods, I have violent nightmares. In a recurring one, I have died as a little girl. Darkness has settled over the Humlegården park in Stockholm and I'm crouched down, shovelling black earth out of my grave with my bare hands. It's night-time and I'm alone in the park. The hole in the ground grows. Down in the dirt, I glimpse a green nightgown with white flowers, a lock of blonde hair, the handlebar of my doll's pram from BRIO. I'm alive and grown up, yet the girl's body lies buried in the dirt. What's happened to me? Why did I die?

For as long as I can remember, I have felt different.

I count backwards. Since the age of 18, I have seen six different therapists for individual therapy and three couples or family therapists, been on two different kinds of antidepressants and various anxiety meds, read piles of books and articles about mental illness, and spent a weekend at the psych ward. Nothing has helped. None of what is said or written fits. It's never describing me.

Slowly, a thought has matured in me: It can't be possible that I'm supposed to feel this way. Therapy and medications are supposed to work, aren't they? People go to therapy for a limited period, not their whole lives. I'm not young anymore. I have to finish this.

I try another route to find the clinic, giving way to a large man in a denim vest who is yelling out for change, hurrying my steps without knowing if I'm walking in the right direction. The downtown area seems fluid, as though the streets have shifted every time I turn my eyes in a new direction.

Over the years, I have tried to identify with the most common mental struggles affecting women. I have wondered whether I'm guilt- or shame-driven, self-effacingly preoccupied with pleasing others, a high-achieving good girl racing towards burnout, a perfectionist with an eating disorder who hates her body. Or simply chronically depressed?

No, it's not right. None of it. On the contrary — most of the time I don't care what others think of me. I achieve, but only in areas that interest me. Anything that bores me, I ignore. When it comes to my body, I'm indifferent. In conversations with friends, I sometimes try to pretend to care about sugar and exercise — things that women are expected to be interested in — but in truth I eat anything I want. I have never perceived my self-worth to be tied to my body.

And yet this relentless anxiety and debilitating fatigue. Do I have trouble sleeping? Not at all; I'm out like a light every evening.

There has to be a reason.

Finally, I find the entrance to the neuropsychiatric clinic for adults.

The psychologist I'm seeing has a name that I interpret as feminine. I imagine a wise older woman, close to retirement, with reading glasses on a cord around her neck. The kind who stands firmly rooted in her long experience — who has seen it all and doesn't fear anything.

The people in the waiting room look normal. White earphones, sneakers. A man in a light-blue sports jacket is absorbed in his phone. On the tables are mandala books for colouring. I open one. 'It's not a chemical imbalance, it's an imbalance of power,' a previous visitor has scribbled on the title page. 'Neither — it's a dysfunction,' a different handwriting replies. 'But it's still a part of you, so be proud!' a third one points out.

A woman steps up to the front desk to pay for her visit.

'Receipt,' says the guy behind the glass.

The woman looks at him in confusion.

'Do you mean if I need it?' she asks.

A tiny bubble of joy rises inside me. She and I are related. How are you supposed to know what someone means when all he says is 'receipt'? It sounds like a statement, not a question. I have come to the right place. These are my people.

'Clara?'

My psychologist walks up, holding out his hand. He is a small man in hipster clothing. He is younger than me and quite good-looking. Damn it. Behind his back in the corridor on the way to the consultation room, I feel like a mental case. A particularly difficult one that should be locked up right away.

He explains matter-of-factly how the assessment will proceed. He will interview me and speak to my close family, we will do tests, and I will fill out questionnaires. I say that I'm worried about not being believed. The friends with whom I have shared my suspicions about autism have all replied: 'Not *you*!'

'I know how to behave. I'm a grown woman and I've practised all my life. I'm really good at keeping up a front,' I warn.

He chuckles.

'There's no point in putting up a front here.'

Afterwards, I google him. He runs a podcast about geek culture.

I have been waiting for over a year to start the assessment, and it wasn't until I called up the Patient Advisory Committee that it became my turn. I want to be evaluated within the public healthcare system, not through a private clinic. The risk that I will wonder afterwards if I have bought my diagnosis must be eliminated. This shall be done right.

I want to speak truthfully and honestly, so ahead of the next meeting with the psychologist I draw up a list of my difficulties lest I forget something:

> I'm the kind of person who puts too much faith in words.
>
> I don't pick up on subtext.
>
> I don't realise that people might be lying.
>
> When I speak, my words fall to the floor and lie there. I feel an enormous sense of powerlessness at not being able to make myself understood.

I'm often angry with others because they don't understand what I mean.

I keep in touch with more people than I have the energy for.

I like to talk about the same thing for a long time, and don't like conversations that jump too quickly between topics.

I struggle with eye contact.

I have a hard time working with others, because no one thinks like me. I become impatient with other people's slowness.

I don't like repeating myself. I have already said what I wanted to say once — that should be enough.

In social situations, I mimic and put on an act. I'm scared of people.

I can't handle abruptly switching between roles, such as my parenting and professional roles, being torn between worlds.

I can't find a balance between the children's needs and my own. I run myself into the ground.

I can't handle being interrupted — for example, speaking on the phone with someone who wants something other than what I'm thinking in the moment.

I don't like changing plans.

I get tired quickly and need a lot of breaks.

I have a few strong interests. But I'm uninterested in much.

I constantly feel like I'm not being left alone.

I'm sensitive to sound. I wear sunglasses and earphones at all times.

I'm intelligent in certain clearly defined areas, such as linguistically and theoretically, yet completely incapable in others. I can't do simple maths or follow basic instructions concerning anything practical.

I struggle with routines, such as showering and brushing my teeth. I do it, but there is a resistance. Anything practical or physical requires a great deal of effort.

I have a poor sense of direction, to the extreme. I get lost in the corridors at work, where I walk every day.

I'm all but face blind, unable to recognise people. But I remember everyone's name!

I have a hard time with chitchat, don't know what to say. I want to speak, but I'm tongue-tied.

The gap between outer reality and my inner world is too wide. The two don't connect.

Reading through the list, I want to laugh. Who is this madwoman?

THE AUTISTS

[It's] like being in a transparent box. No one can hear you.
They can see you, but they can't interact with you. You
can bang on the wall, but you can't get out of it. So, it's
very lonely being in the box your entire life.

OLIVIA, PARTICIPANT ON THE REALITY SHOW

LOVE ON THE SPECTRUM

A brain is born. Three weeks after conception, when the embryo is smaller than a millimetre, a groove forms in the future fetus. The groove is covered over and becomes a tube, one end of which expands into a bubble. This little bubble is the beginning of the brain. When a child with autism is born, somewhere along the way the brain has developed differently.

The cause of autism is biological and there is a strong hereditary component. It's a tricky field of research, involving many different genes. Children can inherit a genetic vulnerability to developing autism. But for autism to arise requires a certain amount of genetic differences, so the specific combination of genes is crucial. This also means that not all siblings in the same family necessarily become autistic.

Sometimes such genetic vulnerability doesn't exist in the parents but arises spontaneously in their sex cells or during the fetal stage — though this is less common. Such genetic mutations can, for example, be caused by the immune system overreacting to a viral infection, by stress or trauma in the mother during pregnancy, by brain injury at birth, by the parents' age, or by the child being born extremely prematurely. What's certain is that no one becomes autistic from vaccinations or the environment they grow up in.

A different brain leads to a different way of being and functioning. Autism is not a disease. It can't be trained away, and there is no medication.

Today, so-called 'high-functioning autists' are diagnosed with autism spectrum disorder without intellectual impairment. What used to be known as Asperger's syndrome has, since 2013, been incorporated into the term 'autism spectrum disorder' in the psychiatric diagnostic manual DSM-5. The designation 'Asperger's' is on its way out, but is still used occasionally. The term 'spectrum disorder' reveals that many ways of being and functioning in the world fall under the same umbrella. The autism spectrum is wide and includes people who experience great difficulties and may, for example, be non-speaking, as well as individuals with demanding full-time jobs. The degree of autism is differentiated into three levels indicating how much support the individual needs, where 1 is the lowest.

Autism is relatively new as a term and a diagnosis, but not as an experience. As a condition, it has always been present in humanity. But throughout history, the language to describe autistic people has varied. They have sometimes been referred to as 'withdrawn', 'eccentric', or 'odd'.

Autism cuts across categories such as age, class, gender, and ethnicity. It exists all over the world and expresses itself in similar ways across different cultures.

Autism makes itself known early, even in the first or second year of life, and children with autism grow up to become autistic adults. Despite this, almost all public discussion of neuropsychiatric diagnoses revolves around children and young people. It's as though we think people grow out of it. They don't.

Another, even stronger misconception about autism is that it's a distinctly male condition. The image of the typical autist as a man has long been prevalent in both research and culture. High-functioning autism, or Asperger's syndrome, was seen as a diagnosis for boys. For a long time, girls of average or above-average intelligence weren't even thought to be able to have autism. Such girls were said not to exist.

There are certain widely established conceptions around men with autism, yet the autistic woman remains unknown in our time.

In fiction — films, TV shows, and books — the gifted and socially awkward woman is portrayed as a copy of the male geek, with identical glasses and the same interests.

A neurodivergent woman who can write a doctoral thesis in theoretical philosophy but has to stop and think when slicing a loaf of bread, who collects teacups and has to recuperate for a day after seeing friends, who loves animals but avoids eye contact is a rare figure in the public consciousness.

This book is about her. About women with high-functioning autism.

The term 'high-functioning' is controversial. Its opposite would be 'low-functioning'. If I had an intellectual impairment, I wouldn't want to be designated as low-functioning.

Being classed as high-functioning doesn't make you a savant, with the ability to memorise never-ending series of playing cards like Dustin Hoffman's character in the film *Rain Man*. It simply means that you are of average, or above-average, intelligence and that you can hold down a job and maintain a relatively well-functioning life.

At the same time, these categories are needed to account for the many different faces of autism. The research quickly gets thorny if we use the same broad concept — autism — to designate varying degrees of difficulty. The term 'high-functioning' may also contribute to removing the stigma around autism and counteracting the prejudice that all autists have an intellectual impairment, because that is not the case. Between 1 and 1.5 per cent of the world's population are autists. Roughly 75 per cent of them are of so-called 'normal' or 'high' intelligence.

More than 100,000 Swedes have autism.

More than five million Americans have autism.

In order to be diagnosed with autism spectrum disorder, a person has to fulfil seven criteria. These include deficits in social communication and interaction, for example in adapting one's behaviour to different settings. The individual must also display a limited range of behaviours and interests, perhaps relying heavily on routines, struggling with change, having strong special interests, and being hyper- or hyposensitive to sensory input. These symptoms must have existed since early childhood and negatively affect their day-to-day life.

The diagnostic criteria are generally formulated in terms of deficits, yet autism is simply a different way of functioning. While autism itself is a condition with biological causes, the *idea* of autism is a social construct. If the norm hadn't been based on the brains of the majority, autism as a label wouldn't exist. Autism challenges established dichotomies such as presence and absence, silence and speech, normal and abnormal, obstacle and asset.

Mentalisation — the ability to perceive one's own and others' thoughts and feelings — functions differently in autists. For an autist, reading and interpreting body language and facial expressions require active thought processes. What others do automatically, the autist must do intellectually. This can make it harder to draw conclusions about other people's intentions. But a person who interprets communication literally and fails to recognise hidden meanings also tends to be honest, with a strong sense of justice.

People with autism receive and process information differently. Autists find it easier to see and focus on details than totalities. People who aren't autists often do the opposite; they take in the big picture, but might miss the details.

Being an autist also means struggling with goal-oriented behaviour. Starting and finishing things can be difficult, and autists like to use the same strategies or do the same thing in different situations. Neurotypical individuals — more specifically, those who do not have autism — can flexibly switch strategy based on the demands of a new situation. Their day-to-day activities, such as cooking or toothbrushing, often happen by routine and don't require much thinking or energy.

Autists often have a so-called 'uneven cognitive profile'. An autist can be very competent in one area, while experiencing great difficulties in another. In many situations, focusing on details, having special interests, and being stubborn can be strengths. The hardest part is usually all the other stuff: social interaction, relationships, and everyday life.

Autistic traits can be found in about one out of five people. But to be diagnosed with autism, a person has to fulfil all seven criteria. In common parlance, you might sometimes hear the comment 'everyone is a little autistic'. But that's a misconception. If you are an introverted person who doesn't meet the remaining criteria, you are not autistic — simply withdrawn.

§

Back in Hagsätra, I'm sitting across from the psychologist in the consultation room at the clinic. It's our second session. It's late in the summer, and the sun casts shadows on the pine table between us. Through the open window comes the sound of a jackhammer drilling into at the asphalt on the other side of the motorway.

The diagnostic assessment is about to begin. The psychologist takes out a bundle of self-report inventories. They are a little antiquated in their view of autism, he says apologetically, but can still offer a good indication. The point of the questionnaires is to evaluate the degree to which various statements apply to me. I'm supposed to fill them out before our next visit.

The psychologist is aware that the examples in the questions are based on men. On the children's forms, they have now added questions to better target girls, but these are still missing on the adult version. He says that we can go through my answers when I'm ready, in case I find anything to be unclear.

At home, I jot down angry notes in the margins.

Do I like playing boardgames? No, not in particular. But I realise it's probably expected of me as an autist.

I usually notice number plates on cars. No, definitely not — I'm not the least bit interested in cars. 'Male-oriented', I note in the margin.

I'm fascinated by numbers. No.

I don't particularly enjoy reading fiction. Yes, I do actually.

Do I like gathering information about different categories of things, such as car makes and different kinds of trains? No. Why this never-ending fixation on vehicles.

Do I enjoy social gatherings and meeting new people? I realise I'm expected to be leaning towards a no. But I usually find that stuff pretty exciting. Sure, it does sap my energy enormously, I often get into misunderstandings with others, and I have to rest for a long time afterwards — but I have never been a complete loner. I have always had friends.

I envision the person whom the questionnaire is aimed at: an anaemic male gamer who rarely leaves his apartment, collects soda cans, can solve a Rubik's cube in under a minute, and monotonously drones on and on about the Cretaceous period. I think about the characters in TV shows like *The Big Bang Theory* and *Atypical* and other male geeks in popular culture.

The self-report inventory assesses me based on how masculine I am.

THE INVISIBLES

I feel invisible and exposed at the same time. Do you feel
that way, too?

@DAISYCAKE65 ON INSTAGRAM

The sculpture stands hidden between two tall oaks. It depicts a huddled
child without a face. The child is crouching with its arms close to its
chest.

Inside the grove of trees in the park in Vidkärr, Gothenburg, the
autumn leaves are stained with rust and the rain drizzles quietly. A naked
branch reaches out above the child's head, which is turned upwards, as
though looking at something in front of it. The child is at the mercy
of an invisible, all-powerful figure. As I tower before little *Alone*, I am
transformed.

This was once the location of one of Sweden's biggest children's
homes. Vidkärr Orphanage was inaugurated in 1935 with room for 200
children from the age of one to 16. These children's homes are a stain on
the national conscience.

When Margareta Ryndel's *Alone* was unveiled in 1988, ten years after
the orphanage shut its doors, the sculpture was accompanied by a plaque

reading: 'In 1935–1976, many children were met with love and care at Vidkärr Orphanage and were given a good start in life.' The grown children objected. They spoke of physical abuse, neglect, violations, forced feeding, and sexual abuse. One doctor and two headmistresses were identified as particularly culpable. The plaque was removed.

Over the years, thousands of Swedish children lived at Vidkärr, and many were subjected to a suffering as systematic as it was meaningless. In a recurring punishment, children were locked up and isolated for up to a week, or forced to shower in ice-cold water. The buildings were surrounded by a six-foot fence with barbed wire. These children had been placed at the orphanage by the Child Welfare Board in Gothenburg.

Today, all the buildings are gone — except one. But the grown children haven't forgotten. *Alone* has been decorated as though the sculpture were a grave. On the ground, among the wet leaves, someone has left a hand-painted pink heart with the words: 'What's the meaning of life if you are forced into a destructive, crushing loneliness?'

The buildings in the area house preschools, care homes, and psychiatric services for children and adolescents. From *Alone*, I walk along the trail through the park grove. On the chain-link fence outside the preschool, the children's rubber boots have been hung in a line. There are no children in the playground; inside, the lights are off.

From the corner of my eye, I see a wooden face appear to my right. It's an overturned log that, like a giant, has fallen headfirst and been left lying under a young maple. On the tree giant's back, three words have been carved in Latin: *Contra spem spero*. 'Against all hope, I hope,' said the artist Hieronymus Bosch.

Is it a vain hope, a hope against better judgement? Or is it a message about the capacity to endure and never give up? The artist who has created the tree giant leaves an ambiguous message for anyone following the path from *Alone* towards the place where Vidkärr Orphanage once stood.

The boxlike, off-white building — all that remains of the orphanage — is now a hospital school for children and young people with serious psychiatric problems in full-time care. The building is so shabby that it's difficult to grasp it is still in use. Hanging in the windows are broken blinds and washed-out curtains; on the top floor, school desks have been stacked against the glass. But inside one of the classrooms the light is on, and I glimpse a computer and a wall clock.

One autumn day in 1989, the junior doctor Svenny Kopp arrived here, at the house with the white facade, to start working for the reputable child psychiatrist Christopher Gillberg.

Kopp had met Gillberg at a medical conference, where he had asked her to join the child-neuropsychiatric project he was about to launch. At the time, he was busy putting together his team.

Kopp became one of the first doctors to join the project, and her task was to examine children whose parents had sought help when they were just three to four years old. Children came from all over Sweden to the former orphanage in Vidkärr.

'These were children with very serious mental impairments,' Kopp says when I visit her at her present place of work, the Gillberg Neuropsychiatry Centre, on Kungsgatan in Gothenburg.

The children were severely autistic and some of them engaged in self-harm, lacked language, and had severe intellectual disabilities. All kinds of children were assessed. Most of them were not 'of normal intelligence', as it was known back then, but there were also some who were.

The way the children were assessed, on the cusp of the 1990s, was similar to today's assessments — only with the difference that, back then, doctors didn't have access to the autism-specific tools ADI and ADOS. Instead, they made a psychological assessment of the children, observing them in and outside of school, assessing their speech and motor skills, and speaking to their parents.

The majority of the children were boys, but there were also many girls. The parents seeking help were worried that the girls were different

— in their capacity for language as well as developmentally. Among the children with severe cognitive difficulties, the gender distribution was fairly even. But among the children of so-called 'normal' intelligence, there was only one girl for every ten boys. Suddenly, the girls were nowhere to be found.

Even though the girls were assessed the same way as the boys, they were rarely given an autism diagnosis.

'It doesn't feel like autism to me' was a sentiment often expressed, explains Kopp. The doctors didn't think the girls fit the mould. Instead, the girls were given other, less-specific diagnoses — such as semantic-pragmatic disorder or learning difficulties.

Why are there no girls of normal intelligence with autism, the medical science of the time asked itself. The explanation, doctors decided, was that girls must have a more extensive brain injury, a profound intellectual disability, before they could develop autism.

And thus, the idea that girls had to have a greater neurological injury and cognitive impairment than boys in order to be diagnosed with autism had been established. There were no girls with high-functioning autism. But Kopp didn't buy it.

Being a woman herself was pivotal to her scepticism, she says today — 40 years later. She saw that women's autism was a blind spot for her male colleagues, and found it provoking.

'I thought it seemed so utterly stupid that girls couldn't be of normal intelligence while also being autistic. Why should autistic girls have a more severe intellectual disability than boys? I didn't understand the explanation. Why would that be the case?'

Kopp had been an active member of the feminist movement, getting involved in the Women's House in Stockholm, and having a feminist perspective since her mid-20s.

But her colleagues thought differently. Many doctors and psychologists at the child psychiatric clinic based their assessments of the girls on a feeling; the girls 'didn't seem to have autism'.

'This was during the psychodynamic era, when everything was the parents' fault,' says Kopp.

As recently as in the 1980s, psychology students were taught that what caused autism in children was an unfeeling mother. Neuropsychiatric diagnoses were not established in the collective consciousness, and within child psychiatry the prevailing view was that autism and ADHD did not have biological causes. Instead, psychiatrists sought the explanation in the child's home life, focusing on family relations and family therapy. In the 1990s, the psychodynamic approach still dominated.

But Kopp didn't give up. She gathered the girls at the clinic in Gothenburg and examined them carefully. All but one were of so-called 'normal' intelligence. Kopp followed the screening instructions carefully, without mixing in any feelings as to whether the girls 'seemed' autistic. It turned out that all of the girls fulfilled the criteria for autism.

'When you ceased questioning on the basis of emotion and were straight-up square about it, the results did show that the girls were autistic. If we are thorough in our assessments, ask the right questions, and understand the impairment, the girls become visible,' says Kopp.

There was, and is, a big difference between having boys and girls as patients, she says. Even though autistic girls could be difficult to connect with, they had a softer presence and 'a girly daintiness'. They didn't dominate the room like the boys did.

'A boy has to be appeased if you're going to get him on board — he won't appease you. He doesn't care about you. Boys do as they please, they're little lords even at the age of three. Girls don't require as much work, even if they have autism,' Kopp says.

'A girl will stand timidly and wait, regardless of whether she has autism or not. Unless she's extremely hyperactive — but even then, she won't display the same dominating behaviour as the boys.'

Yet even though the girls behaved differently when interacting with doctors, their parents spoke of exactly the same symptoms as in the boys. The girls struggled with change, couldn't shower, couldn't handle brushing their teeth, were hypersensitive to sound, had big outbursts at home, slept poorly, and had no friends. These were lonely girls. They didn't play with dolls; instead, they cut them to pieces or just sat there combing the doll's hair. Some of them liked to sort coloured pencils into lines.

'I've never believed that parents come to a child psychiatrist over trivial things,' Kopp says emphatically. 'It's not exactly fun. I've believed that they come because of something real, and I've always thought that it's my duty to find out what. That's my attitude.'

Together with her boss, Christopher Gillberg, she wrote the first scientific article arguing that there were more autistic girls than previously believed. Gillberg and Kopp emphasised that not all autism looks like the kind observed in boys. The year was 1992 and the article was published in a new European journal of child psychiatry. Over time, it has received an incredible amount of attention and citations.

But in the 1990s, it was still controversial to give a neuropsychiatric diagnosis to children. The resistance against the notion that their problems had biological causes was strong.

'The children were all said to have dysfunctional family relationships or a stress reaction, or something along those lines,' says Kopp. 'That problems may arise in family relationships because of the child's difficulties, I can understand. But they're not the cause. "Teenage troubles" was a diagnosis the girls could get. What is that? You know, it would drive me insane.'

A spark lights up in Kopp's eyes, where we are seated in her office at the Gillberg Centre. Her dog peers at us from its place in the corner.

'Christopher Gillberg is the one who has saved the Nordic countries from psychodynamic doom,' she says. She pauses. 'If it weren't for him, I wonder what would have happened to child psychiatry. He had read so very much and understood early on that he needed contacts abroad. There, people maintained a different perspective and intellectual level.'

According to the psychodynamic approach, the children's problems could be solved with various forms of therapy. Kopp emphasises that aspects of such treatment could be sensible. For example, counsellors had a meaningful role to play in supporting parents. But the approach also meant that a child with bowel incontinence could end up going to play therapy from the age of five to nine, without any effect whatsoever. Yet the therapy continued, because the doctors were convinced that the method was correct. Aggressive boys were made to stand at workbenches and bang on chunks of wood to liberate themselves.

Holding therapy, which consisted in holding a screaming child until it gave up, occurred in child psychiatry. It was devastating for autistic children, some of whom experience physical touch as agony. Gillberg was against the method from early on.

Kopp, who was initially psychoanalytically oriented, says that it took her two years to change her own thought patterns.

'I fully understand that it's not easy.'

Child psychiatrists of the time who were interested in the role of the brain had to start up or seek out new clinics. Kopp became head of a child and adolescent psychiatry clinic where they decided to work with autism diagnoses for children. She got the staff on board, they were trained in new examination procedures, and the children were assessed. The proportion of children who received a neuropsychiatric diagnosis at the clinic rose sharply, from 24 to 45 per cent over five years' time. In parallel, she continued her research on girls.

Without Gillberg's support, Kopp believes that her research would have been impossible. He was broad-minded and curious and he encouraged her. But she still ran into resistance in the research community.

At my next visit to the psychologist in Hagsätra, I hand in my completed questionnaires. We go through them together and I quibble over semantics, but he is patient. He says that I can switch out the examples that mention cars, games, and trains for something else in my mind. It doesn't matter which interests I have had. What matters is getting an idea of the intensity with which I have pursued them.

Intellectually, I understand that he is right. But in that case, why even include examples in the first place, I think sourly. After all, autists are known to interpret everything literally. If it says 'car', I don't assume that it might also mean 'music'.

He asks about my childhood, and I recall learning everything there is to know about birds. During break time in primary school, I would sit in the library memorising the species in my bird book. I never had any use for this knowledge where I lived, in Östermalm, central Stockholm. There, we only had house sparrows. But I fantasised about the albatross with its mighty wingspan and dreamt of travelling to Greenland to see the puffins with their peering eyes and striped beaks. I read the book *Jonathan Livingston Seagull*, wishing I was the indefatigable seabird who stubbornly continued to practise nosediving from the sky.

I was obsessed with reading, devouring several books a day, hiding them in my desk at school and re-reading my favourites so many times that I knew them by heart. If I was invited over to a friend's house with a well-stocked comic-book shelf, I would sit down on the floor and read, forgetting to talk to her.

The psychologist asks whether I opened up and shared about myself with others.

'I've never really talked about myself. But I can't recall anyone asking, either.'

'Not even at home? About what happened at school and things like that?'

'No. My parents didn't ask much. But I didn't feel like I had anything to say, either. I kept a diary, instead.'

§

I can remember three sounds from the home I grew up in. The first is silence. The second is booming classical music. The third is the creaking of the hardwood floor as someone moves through the apartment. There is barely any speech, no voices talking. Dad reads in his chair, Mum in her bed. She works there, in bed, in her nightgown and surrounded by piles of open books. Sometimes she speaks on the phone with her sister or a girlfriend, but in such a muted voice that I don't realise there is a conversation going until I open the door to the bedroom that she has closed on herself. Sometimes I hide under a table and write down everything she says in the phone call, but afterwards I can't make sense of my own notes.

When she comes out, she heats up dinner in the oven. Dad gets home late from work, but it's Friday and that means a fancy meal Mum has picked up at the covered market: thick, tender pieces of meat with bearnaise sauce. At Mum's 50th birthday party, Dad gives a speech where he says that she is the only woman he knows who buys ready-made roast potatoes. Then he walks over and kisses her on the cheek.

On Fridays, Dad brings home wine. It's his job to go to the liquor store before the weekend. Mum wants him to serve her at the dinner table, but he will often lose himself in some story and forget to top up her drink. She taps lightly on the side of the glass. His hand trembles as he pours, spilling a few drops on the tablecloth. Mum sighs. She hates stains. But a moment later, the whole thing is forgotten; they have moved into the living room and are sitting around the coffee table listening to Italian opera.

'Could I have some more piss?' Mum giggles, holding out her empty glass towards Dad for some more white wine.

I can feel the anger well up inside me, clogging up my throat. I don't like it when she does that — when she uses the words incorrectly. She calls almost nothing by its right name. Everything has been reorganised along her own associations, and she has decided the rules for what things should be called all on her own without consulting me. It takes me time to interpret the true meaning of her words. 'Marbles' means money, 'the old wagon' is the car, and 'cow secretion' is milk. The latter I understand to be a joke from her father, who is from Gothenburg. She speaks in a jumble of slang, expletives, difficult words, and quotes that sound old. If I complain too much, she replies 'such is life' or that it isn't meant to be enjoyed, it's meant to be suffered and endured. Someone named Schopenhauer has said so.

Sometimes we have guests over: other married couples, variously addressed as justice, professor, or dean. On such occasions, I understand that my mother is funny.

'Are you wearing your lawsuit again?' she says as they take off their coats at the door. They laugh.

Around the dinner table lies a muffled murmur, but Mum's voice breaks through it and I hear her say something that sounds like the crack of whip. There is a moment's silence, then the guests are roaring with laughter.

I lie on my bed listening to the sounds from the dining room. They remind me of *The Cosby Show*. I finger a book on my nightstand, the one that fills me with quiet dread. It's a collection of folktales containing the story of the burning hand — about the two men dressed as women who arrive at an inn late at night and light a fire on a dead man's hand. I crack open the book and peek inside the story about the maid who desperately tries to quench the fire. But the more water she throws on the severed hand, the taller the flames grow. The magical powers of the hand numb the guests at the inn, who drift off to sleep. I tuck away the book and close my eyes, so I won't have to see the face that is taking shape on the wall.

And the hand burned and lulled the people at the inn into a sleep as though they were dead, so deep they could not be woken.

§

The psychologist taps away on his computer. Then he looks up.

'Right. One follow-up question here is whether you usually feel a need to share about your experiences with others. Or is that not so important?'

'Unless something out of the ordinary has happened, I don't think I have anything to say. I don't know what that would be, exactly.'

I'm unsure of whether I have understood the question.

'Is it the function of giving information that is of interest, or could the function be something else?'

'You need to have something to say. And perhaps that means something unusual has happened, or that you have an exciting thought. There has to be *something*.'

'But that wasn't the question precisely. Rather, it's whether you usually feel a need to share your experiences with others? Whether that's a need you have?'

'No, no it's not.'

'So then you're only doing it as part of an act? Because you're "supposed to", expected to?'

'Yes. I imagine that everything exists within me, and that is enough.'

HOLY FOOLS
AND REFRIGERATOR
MOTHERS

'Do you imagine that you saw the king as a father, and the
queen as a mother?'
'They're just pieces.'

CHESS CHAMPION BETH HARMON IS INTERVIEWED

IN THE DRAMA SERIES *THE QUEEN'S GAMBIT*

On a September day in 1731 in the French countryside, just outside
the village of Songy, a group of farmers noticed strange sounds coming
from an apple tree. Up in the canopy, they saw the contours of what
appeared to be a wild animal. It wasn't until the farmers managed to
coax the creature down onto the ground that they discovered it was a
young woman. She was covered in dirt and dressed in rags and animal
hides. Instead of speaking, she emitted loud cries. The farmers gave her a
dead rabbit. With a few swift motions, she flayed it and devoured it raw.

Legend named her the 'Wild Girl of Champagne'. She had survived alone in the woods for a decade, where she had caught fish and hunted birds and frogs. She was said to run incredibly fast and have exceptionally sharp vision.

For more than 250 years, the story about the wild girl was considered a myth. But thanks to persistent archival research, in the beginning of the 2000s evidence was found that proves the story is true. She did exist. Researchers traced her birth to circa 1712 near modern-day Wisconsin in the United States and found that she had belonged to the Native American population and been sold as a slave to a French woman.

How the girl ended up in France is not certain, but she is believed to have been aboard a ship that was quarantined in the port of Marseille after an outbreak of the plague. No passengers were allowed to leave the ship, yet the nine-year-old girl escaped into the Provençal forest. And thus began her decade-long solitude.

After the Songy farmers found her, she was sent to a hospital in Paris and given the name Marie-Angélique Memmie Le Blanc. She moved to a convent where the nuns taught her to read, write, and speak French. Towards the end of her life, Le Blanc lived in Paris among influential friends, including the Duke of Orléans — but she never learnt to appreciate cooked food. The sales of a pamphlet in which she spoke about her life brought her some income. She also received support from the French queen. Le Blanc died in 1775, at the age of 63.

Western history is full of stories about 'feral children' who have survived alone in nature before being brought back to civilisation and becoming subject to scientific interest. Up until the 20th century, these stories were almost exclusively about boys: Peter the Wild Boy from Hamelin; Dina Sanichar from Bulandshahr, who is said to have inspired the character of Mowgli in Rudyard Kipling's *The Jungle Book*; Victor of Aveyron; and Kaspar Hauser, who turned up in Nuremburg in 1828 and was later murdered. Marie-Angélique Le Blanc is the female exception.

The background to why these children were expelled from the family sphere was that they exhibited traits we would today refer to as autistic. All of them lacked human language when they were found. And while some of them eventually learnt to speak, Le Blanc was one of the few feral children who also learnt to read and write.

Contemporaneous interest in these wild children ran high. They were seen as fascinating curiosities and, around them, romantic myths were woven about noble savages and the higher truth of animals and nature. The French naturalists admired the 'natural' soul of a man who may have been ignorant and wild, but also pure, true to himself, and free of hypocrisy.

In reality, these children had often been abused before they were abandoned, and the civilisation to which they were returned labelled them as imbeciles. They were seen as immune to culture, which was set in contrast to the nature in which they had lived isolated.

Autistic people have always existed, but autism as a concept wasn't born until the early 1900s. The history of neurodivergence reflects the views and perceptions that have surrounded people whose brains develop differently, and who thus have certain shared ways of being in common. It touches on questions of knowledge production, seeing, language, and awareness.

The earliest known descriptions of autism date back to the 13th century and refer to the Italian monk Brother Juniper, one of the Grey Friars in St Francis's following. Brother Juniper was, so the sources say, very caught up in details. He interpreted all communication literally, which led to repeated misunderstandings between him and the other brothers of the order. On a pilgrimage when Brother Juniper was being greeted by a procession in Rome, he fixated for hours on a swing — until the welcome party finally tired and left.

Religious sources show that, even then, an awareness existed that certain individuals possessed a specific combination of traits, such as repetitive interests, literalness, being detail-oriented, and struggling to grasp social expectations.

Historically, Christianity has viewed people with certain unconventional behaviours as holy fools. These have been autists, people with epilepsy, and social outcasts of all kinds. A holy fool was considered to be closer to Christ than others, and lived by his own rules. He could be a person whom Christ spoke through directly. Some holy fools were mute; others spoke in riddles. They could say just about anything to anyone, regardless of social convention, making them both admired and feared. Their peculiar manners weren't necessarily interpreted as madness, but rather as holiness.

The professor of Slavic languages and literature Horace Dewey — who had an autistic son himself — has identified what he considers to be signs of autism in 16th-century Russian descriptions of holy fools. In the article 'The Blessed Fools of Old Russia', Dewey and his co-author Natalia Challis study some 30-odd holy fools, all of whom were canonised by the Russian Orthodox Church. They write of St Basil the Blessed, who gave name to St Basil's Cathedral in Moscow's Red Square. Basil, who was born around the year 1468, was a cobbler's apprentice who found God and, in true Robin Hood–fashion, began to steal in order to give to the poor. It is said that Basil often walked around naked in wintertime, weighed down by chains and indifferent to his own needs, such as hunger and sleep. He eventually gained great influence over the first tsar of Russia, Ivan the Terrible, criticising him for his cruelty and flagging attention during worship.

Case reports of boys and men with autistic traits recur throughout the early modern period and into the 19th century, while girls and women are conspicuous by their absence. One rare exception is the British physician John Haslam writing in 1809 about a two-year-old girl who had lost the power of speech after recovering from smallpox.

During the first half of the 20th century, child psychiatry began to take shape as a field of study, and the interest in children with aberrant behavioural patterns grew. Yet early autism research focused solely on boys — leading the diagnostic criteria to be adjusted to behaviours typically coded as male.

The Austrian paediatrician Hans Asperger is usually credited with the discovery of the syndrome later named after him. In 1944, he published an article titled '"Autistic Psychopathy" in Childhood'.

Asperger's early observations were based on four boys he had met. He wrote that the boys suffered from an empathy deficit, struggled to form friendships, made one-sided conversation, were absorbed in their special interests, and moved awkwardly.

Shortly after the end of World War II, Asperger became head of the paediatric clinic in Vienna, where he remained for two decades. With time, he noticed that some of the children he treated went on to become very successful in their professional lives — thanks to their special interests. He called them 'little professors'. One of his patients, Fritz, became a professor of astronomy; another was the Austrian author and Nobel laureate Elfriede Jelinek. As a child, Jelinek used to run from room to room in the family's apartment for hours, getting on her mother's nerves. When she was six years old, her mother brought her to see Asperger.

'Yes, I was an Asperger patient,' Jelinek says in an interview from 1995. 'Not an Asperger autistic, though indeed not far off.'

Asperger concluded that young Elfriede needed an appropriate outlet for her inner tension — which later came in the form of music and writing.

In the same interview, Jelinek calls her mother's decision to subject her to various therapeutic treatments and isolation in their apartment 'a crime'.

'Instead of sending me out to play in the company of kids my age, my mother sent me into the company of severe neurotics and psychopaths.'

In the 1970s, Asperger's early studies were rediscovered by the British psychiatrist Lorna Wing, who coined the term 'Asperger's syndrome'. Wing had an autistic daughter herself — Susie — and came to dedicate her professional life to autism research. She developed Asperger's findings further and published her own case studies. In 1994, Asperger's syndrome became an officially recognised diagnosis.

In 2018, the historians Edith Sheffer and Herwig Czech independently of each other presented evidence that Hans Asperger had collaborated with the Nazis during World War II and been complicit in sending dozens of disabled children to their deaths at the feared Am Spiegelgrund clinic, as part of the Nazi euthanasia program. From 1940 to 1945, 800 children were murdered at Am Spiegelgrund.

Asperger was never a member of the Nazi Party, but of several organisations close to it. He openly supported forced sterilisation and was awarded career opportunities by the Nazis as thanks for his collaboration. All the while, he posed publicly as an opponent of Nazism and continued to work as a respected doctor until his death in 1980.

This new knowledge about Asperger sent shock waves through the autism community. But by 2018, Asperger's syndrome had already been incorporated into the term 'autism spectrum disorder' — so the debate about whether the name of the diagnosis should be changed never gained much force.

Early autism researchers tried to answer the question of what caused the behaviour in autistic children. Was the cause biological or psychological — nature or nurture? Were the children born autistic, or had they become so due to their environment?

They went with the psychological explanation. In parallel with Asperger, the American physician Leo Kanner worked on similar research in the US. When Kanner met with mothers and children in the 1950s, he thought he noticed an aberrant behaviour in the mothers. He perceived them as cold towards their children, and drew the conclusion that this conduct had made the children screen out the world and go into isolation. It was thus the mothers' fault that their children had become autistic, Tanner reasoned. The thought that the mothers might have autism themselves — meaning the cause could be biological — didn't occur to him. Today, it doesn't seem like too wild of a guess to suggest that many of these mothers were autistic, too, and that Kanner mistook their behaviour for cold-heartedness.

The research into autism was a product of its time. It developed in parallel with psychoanalysis, where the patient's childhood was of great significance.

Even before Asperger and Kanner's time, however, there had been an important female doctor who sought other explanations. Instead of 'Asperger's', perhaps we ought to speak of 'Sukhareva's syndrome'. For the Russian doctor Grunya Sukhareva had already described autism almost two decades before Leo Kanner and Hans Asperger. In 1924, she met a 12-year-old boy at the clinic in Moscow where she worked. The boy was reticent and moved slowly. He showed no interest in playing, but appeared very intelligent, and preferred the company of adults. In her diagnosis, Sukhareva described the boy as 'an introverted type, with an autistic proclivity into himself'.

The term 'autistic' was new within psychiatry. A decade earlier, the Swiss researcher Eugen Bleuler had coined the term to describe the way schizophrenic patients withdrew from the world. Through studies of more boys with similar behaviour, Sukhareva expanded the term 'autistic', and in 1925 she published an article with her findings.

'She more or less describes the criteria for autism in the current diagnostic manual DSM-5,' says psychiatrist Irina Manouilenko.

I meet Manouilenko in a deserted Stockholm one spring afternoon during the COVID-19 pandemic. She moved to Sweden in the mid-1990s and wrote her doctoral thesis on the biological causes of autism at the Karolinska Institute. She speaks enthusiastically about the possibilities of brain scanning and Grunya Sukhareva's story.

In Russia, Sukhareva is a big name in child psychiatry. But because of Soviet isolation, her discoveries remained unknown in the West. Only a fraction of 20th-century research findings from the Soviet Union were ever translated into languages other than German.

Sukhareva's research on autism wasn't translated into English until 1996, 15 years after her death, when a British psychiatrist stumbled upon her article in German.

Irina Manouilenko believes Asperger may well have read Sukhareva — who in addition to being a woman was also a Jew — and chosen not to cite her work.

In many ways, Sukhareva was before her time. While Asperger believed autism was caused by upbringing and could be cured with therapy, she saw it as a congenital and neurological condition, tied to the development of the brain. She argued that areas such as the cerebellum, the basal ganglia, and the frontal lobe could be involved. Which is exactly what today's brain imaging shows, says Manouilenko.

Sukhareva never believed in Kenner's idea that autism was caused by cold-hearted mothers. Sadly, the notion of so-called 'refrigerator mothers' would remain prevalent in psychiatry for a long time to come. Perhaps these early ideas about autism as caused by parents are what leads us, even today, to speak of autism in children and young people more often and forget about the adults. Despite knowing that autistic children grow up to become autistic adults — that it's a life-long condition.

LOST IN
THOUGHT

Attention, taken to its highest degree, is the same thing as prayer.

SIMONE WEIL, *GRAVITY AND GRACE*

I join a Facebook group for women with autism and post a question about the special interests of its roughly 2,000 members. The answers come flooding in, and two different categories crystallise immediately: animals and creativity. The women in the group paint, crochet, make jewellery, write, dedicate all their time to bunnies, and work as dog psychologists or with Icelandic horses.

The child psychiatrist Svenny Kopp noticed early on in her research that the interests of autistic girls differed from those of boys.

'No girl was interested in explosives or aeroplanes,' she says. 'But they had other interests. Often, there was a social connection. It could be animals or famous people. A great many of them painted and made things. There was a lot of arts and crafts.'

One reason why girls weren't diagnosed with autism as often as boys was that they were thought to lack special interests. For a long time, psychologists didn't consider girls' special interests as 'real', which contributed to making their autism invisible.

'They were blinded by the special interests of the boys. If a girl collected My Little Ponies and had 75 of them, this wasn't seen as a special interest,' says Kopp. 'The male doctors didn't ask about My Little Pony. They were looking for special interests they could identify with.'

The reason, Kopp believes, is that girls have not been valued as highly as boys, but also that there's an unwillingness to admit differences between the genders.

'It's been a taboo to recognise that we are different, that we have different interests and don't quite function the same way.'

On 9 February 2020, in an attempt to capture the zeitgeist, the journalist Kristofer Ahlström writes about his newfound interest in strength training in the culture pages of *Dagens Nyheter*, one of Sweden's biggest daily newspapers. He has become obsessed with every little aspect of muscle strength, and connects his intense interest to differences between the genders. Why is it only men who allow themselves to be utterly absorbed by their interests beyond all sense and reason, he asks, taking himself and his friends as an example.

Really, the text is about the middle-class ennui, consumerism, and manic competitiveness of a few male individuals in Stockholm. But with the help of masculinity researchers offering sweeping statements about the 'image of masculinity', the conclusions in the article are extrapolated to include all men.

'Why is it not as common for women to go *all in* for some narrow interest?' the text asks. In the hunt for an answer, a gender analysis is formulated that makes it sound as though Sweden were still populated by housewives. Because women earn less, the argument goes, they can't afford to buy expensive outdoor barbecue equipment and nutritional supplements, nor do they have the time, since they are still busy running the home.

In the thought-world of the interviewed masculinity experts, 'special interests' is synonymous with hobbies that men engage in. In other words, if you don't care for sports involving expensive equipment, you don't have any interests.

The same day that *Dagens Nyheter* publishes Ahlström's article and declares that men alone tend to lose themselves in their interests, the evening paper *Expressen* publishes a story about 12-year-old Märta Evertsson, who loves hobbyhorses. She makes them herself, one after another, and has now sewn so many that she no longer has room for them at home.

As a special interest, hobbyhorse-making is estimated to engage more than 10,000 people in Sweden, the majority of whom are girls between ten and 18.

In an apartment in Rågsved, a suburb of Stockholm, the walls are covered with pictures of Marilyn Monroe. Two cats are glaring suspiciously from a corner. 'Asperger kitties,' says Carolina Alexandrou, 31, while pouring coffee into two mugs.

She has a tattoo of Marilyn Monroe's face on her upper arm.

'I've always felt drawn to her. She has been my special interest. Sure, she's beautiful and all that. But the things I read about her story — about the things she went through — that was more important. I could relate to so much and identify with the way she felt. She wasn't doing very well mentally. And she wasn't accepted and appreciated for who she really was.'

Carolina's boyfriend, Roberto, is lying on the couch in the living room, looking at his phone. In a few weeks, Carolina and he are going to see a big Marilyn exhibition in Örebro, a few hours away. The tickets were a birthday gift from Roberto.

Carolina herself began to feel anxious around age 11. It took root in her and never went away. As a child, she always felt different.

'There was something about me that I couldn't grasp.'

She didn't fit in among the other girls her own age, didn't have the same interests, and couldn't understand the unwritten rules of the social game. In upper primary school, Carolina began to isolate. She preferred to stay home reading books and didn't bother trying to make friends. She didn't feel at home in the suburbs where she grew up and felt as though she didn't belong in her own family. Her parents could see that something was wrong, but didn't know how to help her. Visits to the psychiatric services as well as the school counsellor led nowhere.

In lower secondary school, Carolina chose a combined ice hockey and arts program, dedicating herself to her big interest: dance. She trained too hard and began to control her food intake.

'I ate very little and was scared of getting fat. If it was meatballs for lunch, I'd tell myself that I could have two, max.'

Carolina lost weight, but none of the adults around her noticed. In school, she suffered from the ruckus and elevated noise level.

'A classroom full of hockey boys — you can imagine. It was a nightmare. I remember trying to get to know new classmates, but afterwards I learnt that they only hung out with me out of pity. I didn't speak like them, didn't use the same slang. They thought of me as immature and childish. I was like a child all the way up until the age of 16. I wasn't the least bit interested in boys until I turned 18, perhaps. I was a Harry Potter fan who stayed home reading.'

Her peers didn't read. Carolina liked letters but struggled with numbers. She had to retake fourth grade and in lower secondary school she didn't pass maths. She had to do a year of preparatory studies before upper secondary school.

After that, she went to a school for the dramatic arts with a focus on music. Carolina found a friend who took her under wing and taught her how to become more social.

'She trained me. I was very reticent, but she made me open up. I didn't know how to speak to people — what I could and was allowed to say. I had a really hard time with jokes.'

Around the same time, she discovered alcohol as an anxiety reliever. For a time, she fell in with the wrong crowd and partied too hard. Her studies suffered and her grades sank.

'Alcohol was like a magic potion that made me more social. Suddenly I could talk to people without feeling anxious and thinking about what I was doing all the time. But then it got destructive.'

The relationship with her new friends petered out, and Carolina was on her own again. She graduated with an incomplete diploma and registered with the Swedish Public Employment Service.

Then began her search for a place and an industry that might suit her.

In the home of Linn Sundberg, in Falköping, in the south-west of Sweden, I count 25 paintings in different shades of green in the boxes she shows me. Linn is an artist and one of her special interests is Nordic folklore. Hanging on the walls of the dusky apartment with sloped ceilings are illustrations by John Bauer; on the tables are groups of trolls, creatures of the forest, and sprites in felted wool; boxes filled with moss are stacked in the corners. In her bookcase, I spot the fairytale anthology series *Among Gnomes and Trolls*.

Linn says that she feels more at home in the woods than anywhere else.

'It's a bit of a weird thing to say, but I've never felt truly human. I've never identified much with other people, I've always felt different and like a bit of an alien. I feel more at home among spirits than in society the way it looks today.'

The colour green calms her and runs as a common thread throughout her art. She has tried using other colours, but always returns to it. Her artistic work helps her regulate her energy and dampens her anxiety and overthinking.

'It's a bit like walking out into the forest and sitting there.'

She creates her green paintings using a method known as 'acrylic pouring', mixing acrylic paint with varnish glue and using silicone oil to achieve different effects as the paint bleeds. In the paintings, it looks as though round cells are opening up. She paints watercolours, too — pictures of little nodules that look like roots. One root is an autist, with a hood pulled up and headphones.

Linn's wood sprites are mixed-media art. She finds her materials cheap on online marketplaces and in second-hand shops, making little creatures out of pinecones, shelves and lamps out of polypores from dead trees, masks out of moss and luminous paint. She sews, too.

She shows me her creatures. The cone people live in the woods, guarding the crown and the throne while waiting for the rightful heir to come. Care has been put into every little detail.

One creature has a jointed body, where the neck has been made out of a kitchen tap and the body has been filled with tinfoil and shaped out of soft polymer clay. The legs and arms consist of foam tubing with metal wires running through it, wrapped in felted wool; the pants have been sewn out of felt.

'It's some kind of creature of the forest. I imagine it running around helping animals caught in barbed wire. And collecting pretty crystals and other useful things in the woods.'

It has a small knife, made of clay wound with floral tape, and a bag with a selenite stone inside. The bag is made of fabric from an old purse that Linn has saved for 12 years.

'I end up hoarding quite a lot of clothes and fabrics because I go through periods when it comes to what I'm comfortable wearing, and this has turned out to be incredibly useful.'

Linn's brain works fast, but she needs help reining herself in.

'I have so many good ideas, but you can't do everything. It can be very stressful having so many thoughts. I have a hard time focusing on things.'

But when she finds her focus, the results can be extraordinary.

She opens her mouth and sticks out her split tongue.

'The anaesthesia wore off on the train between Stockholm and Eskilstuna, and I sat there drooling blood into a napkin. I had a mountain of luggage, it was January, and I couldn't speak, so I couldn't call a taxi, and had to drag my bags through the snow. There was a trail of blood and drool a mile or two from the station.'

Linn met her partner, whom she now lives with, at a mutual friend's house while recovering from her tongue surgery. He sat there making music on his computer while she wrote him notes, drooling blood into a jar.

Linn is doing an internship at an art gallery in town. She partakes in so-called 'daily activities for people with neuropsychiatric diagnoses' — a type of legally regulated, unpaid daytime activity meant to offer stimulation and promote equal living conditions as well as full participation in society — but she does not have a job. It has never quite worked out. Instead, she receives a habilitation allowance from the National Board of Health and Welfare to be able to work at the gallery, which is run by a non-profit. The municipality pays the gallery's rent and provides a small operating grant.

In the past, she used to receive something called activity compensation, which is offered to people under the age of 30. Now, at 31, she is on what is known as 'sickness benefits in special cases'. It's available as an option for those who still need support but where it has not been determined that they are unable to enter the job market.

For periods, Linn is so absorbed by her creative work that she forgets to eat and go to the bathroom. But there are also times when she isn't doing so well. When that happens, she plays video games so she won't have to think.

'Do you know any tales about changelings?' Linn asks me suddenly, as we are standing in front of her collection of *Among Gnomes and Trolls* books. I nod.

'They were children who were thought to have been switched out by trolls,' she continues. 'A child behaves "normally" when it's young. But as it grows older, it starts acting a little strange — and then it's the trolls who've exchanged it for a troll child. Have you ever thought about that in relation to autism?'

In the book *Trolls and Men*, the folklorist Ebbe Schön writes that the tales about changelings in old Swedish folklore allowed people to explain children who were different. The tales were born out of a need to understand why some children didn't develop like others and how they could be cured. Folklore offered a magical explanation, through which parents could process their concern for their child.

Trolls were thought to live in a kind of parallel world, and were used as scapegoats and evil reflections. Out in the woods, you could smell food from their dwellings and hear them call and shout. They were thought to have a troubled and messy family life.

Because trolls could take on human form, there was reason to suspect that strangers one encountered might actually be trolls. According to tradition, the difference between troll and human was revealed in the way they spoke.

There were words that supernatural creatures were thought to shy away from. For this reason, you were meant to pay attention to the speech of strangers. Someone who said 'big hound' instead of 'bear' or used the word 'earwig' instead of 'scissors', you were meant to look out for. People who were creative with language aroused suspicion. In our time, linguistic ingenuity and an ability to make up new words and metaphors is often associated with neuropsychiatric diagnoses.

One of the most terrible things that trolls could do to people was to steal their newborn baby and replace it with their own child. Often, they would strike before the child was baptised, while it was not yet under Christian protection. The parents didn't notice what had happened until much later, when their child didn't develop in a normal way — when it didn't seem able to learn how to either think or speak. Like a cuckoo chick, the changeling would eat the humans out of house and home. The tales describe the little one lying in bed drooling or stirring up trouble in the household. Having 'a short and uncontrollable temper' could be enough for the parents to say that the child was 'completely changed', writes Ebbe Schön.

There were also stories about the incredible physical strength of changelings and how they could prove to be of unexpected help in heavy labour. The young trolls were older than the human children they replaced and sometimes a changeling might accidentally say too much, revealing its true age. In other words, children who were different could be perceived as older than they really were.

Trial records from, for example, the Swedish island of Gotland in the 17th century reveal that parents could be known to abuse their children if they were thought to be changelings. This treatment was sanctioned by custom, which led parents to believe that they were curing their child by beating it.

In the short story 'The Changeling', the Swedish author Selma Lagerlöf, the first woman to win the Nobel Prize in Literature, turns the myth into a cautionary tale. The main characters of the story — a farmer and his wife — encounter a troll in the woods, who steals their child and leaves her own by the side of the road. Even though the farmer's wife knows that the troll baby is not her own, she brings the child home. The neighbours in the area advise her to flog the changeling with a cane, as they believe that beating it will swiftly make the troll mother return and switch the children back. But the farmer's wife cannot bring herself to strike the innocent child. She protects the troll baby from her husband, feeding it frogs and spiders — food that it likes. The farmer and their servants hate the changeling. As the years go by, their entire community turns against the wife, who stubbornly sticks by the young troll. Not even when the changeling accidentally burns down the farm and her husband abandons her does she stray from its side.

Then one day, the farmer meets his real son out in the woods. From what the young man says, the farmer gathers that his son's life with the trolls has been mirrored by that of the young troll on the farm. Every time the farmer treated the troll badly, his own son was treated badly by the trolls. And the other way around: when the farmer's wife showed tenderness towards the changeling, the human child was treated well, too.

The farmer realises that his wife's kindness towards the changeling has saved their son. Because of her ultimate sacrifice — when she renounced her husband for the sake of the young troll — the trolls could free the human child and the changeling could return home. The farmer has his wife to thank for getting their child back. Yet the happy ending to the story also contains the suspicion that the farmer's wife will miss the changeling after he has disappeared from their lives.

The British children's author Beatrix Potter was deeply fascinated by mushrooms. She collected, studied, and illustrated them tirelessly. With microscopic richness of detail, she painted the spores of different kinds of mushrooms and developed her own theory about the way they reproduced. She wrote down her conclusions in an essay and sent it to the Linnean Society of London, who denied her admission for being a woman. Her hopes of dedicating herself to the science of mycology were dashed, but her strong interest in animals and nature stayed with her throughout life. She collected fossils and kept mice, frogs, hedgehogs, and a stuffed, mounted bat in her home.

From the age of 14, she kept a diary written in a secret code she had created herself. As a grown-up, she wrote and illustrated stories with her own pets as the main characters. *The Tale of Peter Rabbit*, for instance, was based on her own rabbit named Peter Piper.

Visitors described her home at Hill Top farm as an outright menagerie. The people around her spoke of a withdrawn and eccentric individual, who took no interest in social intercourse. When a publisher suggested changes to *The Tale of Peter Rabbit*, she had the book printed by her own press.

Potter was perceived as grouchy, and she didn't like children. When Roald Dahl was six years old, he went to visit the 56-year-old Potter, to meet his author idol.

'What do you want?' she asked when she saw the boy in her garden.

'I've come to meet Beatrix Potter,' he said.

'Well, you've seen her. Now, buzz off!' came the answer.

Was Beatrix Potter autistic? The psychiatrist Michael Fitzgerald believes so.

In the middle of the 18th century, an ideal developed in French painting that centred on depictions of frozen moments of absolute concentration. Artists such as Jean-Baptiste Greuze and Jean-Baptiste-Siméon Chardin painted men, women, children, and elderly individuals deeply engrossed in various activities. The people in the paintings could be reading, listening, painting, writing, thinking, sleeping, studying, or praying — sometimes with their back to the observer. They were utterly and completely absorbed.

The women's role in the paintings was often to listen to a man. Sometimes she was sewing or lost in her own reflection.

In the painting *La Lecture de la Bible* (*'Un père de famille qui lit la Bible à ses enfants'*) from 1755, Jean-Baptise Greuze depicts a father reading from the Bible to his devoutly attentive wife and daughters. The father has stopped to contemplate the words he has just spoken; his gaze is turned inwards, his eyes glassy.

Jean-Baptiste-Siméon Chardin's philosopher in the painting *Un*

Philosophe occupé de sa lecture (1753) has also paused to think. Chardin captures the facial expression of a reader contemplating with intensity the meaning of the words he has just read. As an observer, you feel that the philosopher has forgotten both himself and his surroundings. He doesn't notice that we are watching him.

Why did 18th-century French artists want to depict people lost in thought? In his book *Absorption and Theatricality*, the American art historian and critic Michael Fried writes that it was a reaction to the exquisitely decorative and theatrical rococo movement. They wanted to return to serious, moral themes in their art and to the aesthetic ideals of previous eras. There was a longing for a more authentic expression.

The French artists of the 18th century were not the first to paint people in contemplation, but they were consciously consistent, and refined the expression. Most of all, they secularised concentration and fulfilment, which came to be about something other than religious devotion. Chardin moved raptness into the home and other quotidian environments. It was no longer an experience exclusively reserved for church.

This new French artistic ideal was also tied to the emergence of a middle-class audience who wanted to see moral, narrative motifs in art, preferably in environments they could recognise from their own lives. Introspection was rated highly, and elevated attention was a virtue, something good in and of itself.

But most of all, this development marked a shift in the view of the relationship between a work of art and its observer. Through the faraway-looking, occupied figures in the artworks — who refused to meet the observer's gaze, or sometimes appeared to be staring right through them — they denied the observer's existence. The observer was supposed to be absent. For the artists, it was important to avoid the impression that the figures depicted were actors on a stage, putting on a show for the audience.

The artists were creating scenes that neutralised the observer, who was left out. And the audience of the time loved to be ignored. Greuze's and Chardin's artworks were praised to the skies by art critics.

But what lay behind these artists' conscious exclusion of the observer? Was it elitism? No. Paradoxically enough, the intention was the exact opposite — to invite in as many as possible. The idea was for these deeply absorbed figures to inspire the audience to pause, take in the picture, and become lost in it themselves. For the feeling in the painting to rub off.

You might call it a clever trick, like a trompe l'oeil or hypnotic effect, a manipulation to draw the observer into the painting. A bit like when parents of young children read bedtime stories about drowsy animals to put their kids to sleep, in the hope that the yawning rabbit in the story will make the little listener sleepy, too. But there was also a deeper philosophical background to the figures lost in thought in French 18th-century paintings.

Their lack of awareness also makes them lonely. Perhaps it was exactly this effect that captivated the observer, Michael Fried suggests, since that lonely feeling is familiar to almost everyone. But the sight of figures intensely engrossed can also elicit joyful recognition — at least in an autistic observer.

AN ATTACK ON
ALL SENSES

What's that sound. I hear it all the time. It's a voice, we
might call it the voice. The sound of people talking, the
traces of a song. A baseline murmur. The rustle of the
snake in the grass. The soughing of the valves. The white
noise of my own head — A touch of autism might be the
case; either way, a hypersensitivity to sound. On TV, I
see a little boy desperately clasp his arms around his head
when it's too loud; he's making whipped cream wearing
hearing protection. I burst into tears.

KATARINA FROSTENSON, *THE SKULLS*

Today, Chardin's and Greuze's entranced figures might have been
painted wearing big, wireless headphones. But to depict the taciturn
person of our time as deeply absorbed in a screen doesn't have quite the
same effect as the 18th-century paintings.

Screens capture our attention and turn us away from each other. They are used by many to wind down and clear the mind, though we rarely achieve the same concentrated state as the French painters' subjects. As screen users, we are alternately shocked and distracted, jumping quickly between clips and clicks while staging the present on our social-media channels. In the real now, we become both self-conscious and distant. Unlike the people in the image world of the 18th century who forgot their observers, we are extremely conscious of our audience, preoccupied as we are with the way the now will appear in a near future to an anonymous audience on the internet.

The relaxation form ASMR, on the other hand, has been created to absorb its subjects. ASMR is short for 'autonomous sensory meridian response', and refers to euphoric feelings that arise in response to various stimuli. The name was coined by the American behavioural scientist Jennifer Allen in 2010. The sensation of a pleasant tingling along the head and spine has also been described with words such as 'brain massage' and 'spine shivers'. The ASMR effect can be achieved through visual, auditory, tactile, olfactory, or cognitive stimuli. By listening to soft, whispering voices or watching video clips of people slowly doing mundane things such as brushing their hair, the subject comes to relax and feel a sense of wellbeing. It is a drug-free, digital alternative to pharmaceutical sedatives.

A description of an ASMR-like phenomenon can be found in Virginia Woolf's novel *Mrs Dalloway*:

> 'K ... R ...' said the nursemaid, and Septimus heard her say 'Kay Arr' close to his ear, deeply, softly, like a mellow organ, but with a roughness in her voice like a grasshopper's, which rasped his spine deliciously and sent running up into his brain waves of sound which, concussing, broke. A marvellous discovery indeed — that the human voice in certain atmospheric conditions (for one must be scientific, above all scientific) can quicken trees into life!

Woolf grew up around a neurodivergent person herself. Her 12-years-older half-sister, Laura Stephen, was most likely autistic, according to Woolf's biographer Hermione Lee, who bases her assessment on the memoirs of Woolf's family members and the letters they left behind. Laura had a speech impediment, repeated words and gestures, and experienced recurring outbursts of rage. When she was a little over 20 years old, the family shipped her off to an institution.

Despite living under the same roof, Woolf appears to have been frightened and disgusted by her sister's condition, and wanted to distance herself from Laura. In 1915, she wrote scornfully of a group of 'miserable shuffling idiotic creature[s]' whom she had run into, and declared that 'they should certainly be killed'. In what way this autistic presence in her home may have influenced her writing, we can only speculate, but in his book *Representing Autism* the scholar Stuart Murray wonders if Laura's presence might have contributed to the necessity of 'a room of one's own'.

Some believe that Woolf herself had autistic traits, though no one can know for sure. It has been pointed out that she started speaking late, suffered from anorexia, avoided eye contact, and was reserved and withdrawn and intensely preoccupied by her pens.

Autistic people can have such a hard time with certain sensory stimuli, such as loud noises and bright lights, that these give rise to physical pain. Other sensations, like touching certain types of fabric, can feel deeply satisfying. Since far back in history, people have used so-called 'sensory metaphors' — tasting words, hearing colours, or seeing sound — but it wasn't until the 1980s that science could connect these feelings to real, observable activity in the brain.

The neuroscientist Henrik Jörntell at Lund University argues that conditions such as synaesthesia — associating sounds with colours, for instance — is more common among autists. In a young child's brain there are a great many connections, some of which are peculiar, like those running from the ears to the visual cortex. In most people, such peculiar connections are weeded out as the brain develops, but in some they remain. And this, scientists believe, is the basis for synaesthesia.

In her autobiography about growing up with Asperger's, the author Gunilla Gerland describes how, as a child, she experienced everything in colours. The tone of her mother's voice might, for example, be the colour purple.

Personally, I read an exhilarated description of a trip to Venice as 'an attack on all senses' and shudder with discomfort. I'm so sensitive to sound that the wrong noise grates and claws at my insides. Being overloaded with lights and sounds is painful, and I hear everything: the whirring of the projector in the work meeting, the conversations at the back of the bus, the neighbours calling to each other across the courtyard, the metallic clang of the deadbolt as the door unlocks, the children in the street outside the closed window, the muted humming of the fridge. I cannot filter anything out; everything cuts straight through. The sounds can't be shut out, and hearing protection offers only a partial reprieve.

Because I take in every sound, including conversations, I also remember much of what is said. But neurotypical people appear to be insensitive to repetition. They love to talk about the same thing several times and come to the same conclusion over and over again. In contrast, I become impatient; I feel that what is being said has already been dealt with, especially when it comes to things like instructions at work. Repeating oneself in personal relationships so that I may treasure shared memories is another matter. That, I enjoy.

Being a woman with autism means feeling ill-suited for many of the roles that society offers women. I myself can't relate to the expected female obsession with my own body. I'm not in touch with my body. Every month, my period comes as a surprise. And if I ever contract a deadly disease, I won't be going to the doctor until it's too late, because I won't have noticed that I'm in pain.

I don't notice feelings of hunger, and can go long periods without food. Not because I want to lose weight, but because I forget to eat. Eating is primarily something that disturbs and disrupts my thoughts; it requires an effortful shift in focus that I would rather avoid. But I like good food. I eat like a snake — huge portions at few times.

There is a clear connection between autism and anorexia. Research has shown that eating disorders are just over twice as common among adults with autism as in the population at large. Often, autistic individuals don't feel hunger in the same way as others. They are more likely to forget to eat, and an eating disorder can become an outlet for the anxiety and unrest that social alienation brings. For a person with autism, the world is so unmanageable and the experience of a lack of control so overwhelming that they often cling to the minor aspects of their lives that they can control. Their food intake is one of them.

The journalist and author Lina Liman suffered from anorexia for many years before receiving her autism diagnosis. In her book *The Art of Faking Arabic*, she writes about the road to recovery. Greta Thunberg, who was diagnosed with Asperger's as a 12-year-old, also stopped eating for a time before she found her place and purpose within climate activism.

The autist must find her place in the world, where she can turn her diagnosis into something positive and play to her strengths. In my work as a radio producer, I can use my sensitivity to sound and ability to pick up on details. I hear every poor edit and shift in volume. But wearing my noise-cancelling headphones on the crowded metro on my way to work every day, I ask myself whether it's worth it. I would probably do better in some cabin in the woods.

§

'What's the similarity between music and drift ice?' asks the psychologist in Hagsätra.

I have reached the next step in the diagnostic assessment: an intelligence test. The questions are designed to measure my capacity for abstract reasoning.

'Both are in motion?' I try.

'What's the difference between sympathy and apathy?'

It's a shame he didn't say 'ignorance and apathy', I think to myself. If so, I would have answered: 'I don't know and I don't care.' Why do I feel this constant need to entertain him? I really must stop.

'Sympathy means feeling for someone, while apathy is being indifferent.'

The final comparison is the hardest. What's the similarity between a friend and a foe? None at all, I want to say. It's like asking what light and darkness have in common. After some consideration, I finally manage to say something about both being a type of close relationship.

The psychologist says that he doubts I have an intellectual impairment, but an intelligence test is always part of the screening. I try my absolute hardest, keen to impress him in order to make up for all of my silly struggles that we otherwise discuss.

In the different sections of the test, I'm variously asked to draw lines between identical symbols, piece together squares on which triangles have been painted into a bigger pattern, select the correct images to complete a series of puzzles, and list symbols paired with numbers. Everything involving puzzles and pictures goes badly. It has to do with my ability to interpret what different figures represent based on their shapes, colours, and patterns.

'Next, I'll be reading some words,' the psychologist says. 'So listen carefully and tell me what the words are or what they mean.'

'Okay.'

'Let's start with the word "peach".'

'Am I supposed to say "fruit"?'

'I mean, well, you're supposed to say what the word *is* or what it *means*.'

'Yes.'

'You said fruit?'

'Yes.'

'Let's move on to ... scarf.'

'A piece of clothing worn around the neck.'

The psychologist falls silent.

'... as protection or to keep warm,' I add, just to be safe.

He notes something down with his stubby pencil.

'Lunch.'

'A meal in the middle of the day.'

'Passion.'

'A strong, positive emotion. It can be love or an interest that you love, something you feel strongly about.'

'Palpable.'

'Something you can touch or feel, something real.'

'Scolding.'

'A forceful reprimand.'

'Deliverance.'

'Being set free. Palpable ... I think maybe I meant tangible?'

'We can't go back to that one now, I'm afraid.'

'Oh, okay.'

'Let's move on to ... empathy.'

'Being able to imagine yourself in someone else's situation and feel compassion for that person, or understand the other's feelings.'

'Quick-witted.'

'Fast and humorous. The ability to articulate oneself in a way that is snappy, clever, and funny.'

'Contrition.'

'Remorse.'

'Okay. Good. That's done.'

The test moves on to general-knowledge questions. I deliver swift answers to 'Who painted *Guernica*?' and 'Who wrote the novel *Ivanhoe*?', responding '*Sir* Walter Scott' out of pure competitive zeal, as though that would somehow give me plus points — by which I feel briefly embarrassed — and say 'pass' on all questions about things like the chemical symbol for iodine or how to calculate an object's density.

Then the psychologist reads out long series of numbers, which I'm supposed to repeat — in the same order and in reverse. The air in the little consultation room is running out. When it's time for the mathematical questions, he measures the speed of my response with a stopwatch.

'It takes 31 minutes to make two blueberry pies. How long does it take to make 14?'

I have to use all my willpower not to start questioning whether it takes only 31 minutes to make two blueberry pies.

'Anne has twice as many apples as Peter. Anne has 49 apples. How many apples does Peter have?'

'John is waiting in line behind 80 people. He lets ten people cut the queue in front of him. Each minute, three people reach the front of the line. How many minutes does it take before it's John's turn?'

'Could I hear that one again? Six. No, wait! Thirty?'

And finally, it's over. We have covered four cognitive areas: verbal comprehension, working memory, perceptual reasoning, and processing speed. The psychologist wants to know if I used any strategies, like in the memory tests, when I was asked to repeat a series of numbers.

'Sometimes I tried to mimic the sound of your voice.'

'I could hear that a little, actually.'

It's not really the numbers that I remember so much as the sounds, I think to myself afterwards. If I had seen them written down, my results would have been worse.

My score on the intelligence test is uneven. I perform well above average on verbal comprehension and working memory, and around average on perceptual reasoning.

THE
AUTOMATONS

The extreme difficulty which I often experience in
carrying out the slightest action is a favour granted to me.

SIMONE WEIL, *GRAVITY AND GRACE*

As a child, I remember having my own special movement. When I felt
happy or excited, I would squeeze my elbows against the side of my
body, tense my arms, clench my fists, and shake them underneath my
chin. It happened spontaneously, without me thinking about it.

One day in gym class, a boy called my name. When I looked in his
direction, he and several others were sitting on a bench mocking me. I
gathered that there must be something wrong with the movement, and
stopped doing it.

'Stimming', or 'self-stimulation', is a way of expressing emotion.
It can be smelling or touching pleasant things, making certain body
movements, dancing, singing, repeating words, chewing on something,
studying patterns, or listening to sounds. Autists stim in order to process

and balance their sensory experiences.

I tend to finger my lips, and when I'm in deep concentration in front of my computer I sometimes open and close my mouth rhythmically. For a time when I was younger, I used to tap melodies with my teeth if I was home alone.

My hands are constantly having to relearn. There appears to be no memory in them; they can't remember anything.

Certain finicky things, they do know: how to apply make-up to my face, type quickly on a keyboard, braid my daughter's hair, loosen the crown on a wristwatch with a tiny screwdriver, and open the kind of sugar-cube wrapping they have in cafes with that special trick where the two cubes are pulled apart so the paper tears down the middle and each cube ends up in its own little pocket.

My hands most definitely don't know how to massage, cut grass, or pump air into a bike tyre. They can handle tinkering and fiddling, but not chores. Chores aren't the same as tinkering. Chores are all those tasks that must be taken care of, that must be done: the maintenance of things.

Chores are carried out by capable people. I wish I were capable.

'It's as though the objects and the things and the trees — everything — are just calling out to be taken care of. There are chores to do which I don't have the faintest idea of how to approach,' says Katarina Wikars in her Swedish radio show *That Which Got Out of My Hands*.

She is interviewing the author Margareta Lindholm, who in 2010 published the novel *The Forest*, about an elderly pair of siblings who are forced to leave their farm yet stubbornly continue to sow, plant potatoes, clear weeds, and burn grass to the bitter end.

'We are connected to life through our chores,' says Lindholm.

I see what she means, and I like the thought. It's our everyday chores and routines that form the backbone of our lives: the mechanised movements that keep us alive, the repetitions that bring us into communion with eternity and our roots.

'Until we die, we have to busy ourselves with certain chores. And you can't stop simply because you know you're going to die, or because you know that you're moving elsewhere. It's something that is always ongoing,' she continues.

But what about a person like me, who has such a hard time keeping up with certain chores — where does that leave me? As someone estranged from life itself?

'I'm one of those people who likes to always be busy. I get restless,' Lindholm also says on the show.

People — particularly women — often say that. I find it provoking. The feminine contentment at being steadfast and capable.

Personally, I hate doing things all the time, and I never get restless. I'm a master of being bored. I struggle to be near people in constant motion; their unholy roving stresses me out. Why can they never be still? What do they think is going to happen if they sit down for a moment?

Always 'having one's hands full' is considered a virtue, and there is a connection here to that old Protestant work ethic. We even think of our hands as having a need of their own to do things, to be busy. The value judgement is reflected in our language, in the word 'business', from 'busy-ness', which used to have two meanings: a person's occupation as well as the state of being occupied. Today, 'business as usual' is typically a good thing — the labour required for the maintenance of the world as we know it — while to 'have no business' means to have no right. Yet further back, 'business' also signalled a state of anxiety.

There are things that just have to get done. Eating, making the bed, brushing your teeth, showering, cleaning. How can it be so hard?

Autistic people don't use the automatic memory in the brain when carrying out practical tasks. Instead, they engage a part of the brain that solves problems intellectually. Neurotypicals use their automatic memory for things like turning on the coffee maker or the dishwasher. For them, it happens reflexively; they don't have to think about what they are doing. That's not what it's like for me. Every time I need to lock the front door, turn on the oven, chop onions, or fold up the ironing board, the same brief little thought runs through my head: 'How do you do this again?' Often, it feels as though I'm going through the motions for the first time, despite thousands of hours of prior experience.

I wish I was more automatic. I wish I was more like my friends who can invite people over for dinner and stand in the kitchen cooking while making unforced conversation with their guests. To me, it is incomprehensible the way they can chop vegetables all the while they are speaking, asking, thinking, and answering. I don't understand how it works. I never invite anyone over for dinner; it's too much effort. I have to rest for two days afterwards.

Not being able to fend off sensory input, constantly taking in one's entire surroundings, and thinking about every little movement of the body is draining. My perceptive faculties are always in overdrive. I'm incapable of screening out irrelevant sounds, words, and images that invade my world.

I show the YouTube video 'Autism: Bus Ride' to my children in an attempt to explain how it feels. In the clip, a man boards a bus and is immediately attacked by a cacophony of sounds: tyres screaming as the driver pumps the brakes, the huge metal vehicle creaking as it moves, the engine roaring, the driver's radio blaring, the second hand on a watch ticking relentlessly, and the passengers' conversations booming in parallel in the poor man's ears, while the schoolkids at the back holler and carry on and the pensioner in the seat next to him wants to chat. At the next stop, he stumbles off the bus, ready to faint. 'Is that what it's like?' the children ask. 'Yes,' I say. 'But I'm always wearing earphones,' I add, so they won't have to worry.

It will always be like this, but I don't tell them that. I will never become automatic. I will never have access to the same generalised information as they do, brushing their teeth without thinking.

There is a text by the Russian author Viktor Shklovsky that makes it easier to breathe. In it, he warns of the dangers of perceiving the world by routine. If we take in our surroundings too habitually, eventually perception itself becomes automatised. An increased automatisation of perception means 'we save the greatest amount of perceptual effort', which in turn leads us to live a greater part of our life on an unconscious level.

'This is how life becomes nothing and disappears,' writes Shklovsky. Automatisation devours phenomena. He quotes Leo Tolstoy: 'If the whole complex life of many people is lived unconsciously, it is as if this life had never been.' Thus, life slips away.

Habit leaves us numb and robs us of our capacity for awe. Automatised observations allow our souls to slowly petrify, turning us into robots. The cure is art, which increases the complexity of perception, and thereby its duration.

I will never perceive the world habitually, because I am constantly taking in new details. Every day, the streets are new and untrodden. I'm the proverbial goldfish that forgets its aquarium with every new circle that it swims.

I suppose I will have to try to think of it as living a conscious life. At least, I tell myself, I'm no soulless robot, closed off from poetry, art, and religion. It's cold comfort when I lose my way for the thousandth time, when I gather strength to brush my teeth, or when I stand in front of the kitchen fan trying to figure out which button to press.

My endeavour to clear away obstacles in day-to-day life has led to a dependence on strict routines. That's what it's like for many autists. Life becomes easier if it's predictable. I like to eat the same food every day, go to the same island every summer, and I love doing things at a specified hour so I have time to prepare.

§

Elisabet, 77, is a retired professor who, throughout her life, has been forced to find strategies to deal with the demands of living. Instructions for household appliances, phones, and computers have always been near impossible for her to decipher, so she writes her own manuals in a language she can understand.

In her self-authored manual for how to turn on her phone, she writes: 'When unlocking the phone and the nine fried eggs appear, trace a U with your finger.' The fried eggs are the round glyphs representing touch-phone buttons.

If someone calls her on the phone, the instruction reads: 'Press the green button and slide your finger to the right. Speak. End the conversation by pressing the red button, unless your counterpart has already ended the call.' If she wants to turn off the phone: 'Trace a U with your finger if the fried eggs appear.'

Elisabet has similar manuals for the washing machine and the dishwasher, the coffee maker, her speakers, the computer, the TV, and the fuse box. By formulating the instructions in her own words, she makes them intelligible to herself. The idea is her own; she has never sought help for her difficulties. She is an intellectual heavyweight, one of Sweden's most well-qualified researchers in her field. And for 50 years she was married to a man who could support her in the practicalities of life.

Ida Hallin Mellwing is 36 and lives in Valdemarsvik, a small town on the coast of the Baltic Sea. She cleans her bathroom every Monday; every other Wednesday, she cleans the family's aquarium; and every three weeks, she grooms the dogs.

On the wall in their home is a rolling schedule of household chores that she follows. It tells her what to do each day. One day, she dusts; the next, she vacuums. Always a little bit at a time, so the chores don't become overwhelming.

There is always a nappy bag at the ready, even at home, and Ida makes sure to keep dummies everywhere. There is a car dummy, a pram dummy, and a bedroom dummy.

Through living by the schedule and doing everything to avoid stressing about the little things, Ida simplifies her life as a parent of young children. The schedule also doubles as an uplifting receipt of what she has actually managed to do and accomplish each day.

At 25, after suffering from panic attacks and depression, she underwent an assessment that resulted in an autism diagnosis. Throughout her schooling, she had blamed herself, feeling stupid and different.

'I've always been odd. I became a social outcast and had no friends who knew the real me. I felt very lonely.'

When the others talked, Ida tried to be part of the conversation. But whenever she said something, the response was often 'Huh?' Ida says that she struggled to understand why almost no one wanted to hang out with her. When she was younger, she sometimes had outbursts, which she thinks many were deterred by. She had a strong sense of right and wrong and of justice, and could end up in a conflict if someone behaved badly. She couldn't stand classmates who were disruptive or made annoying sounds, and could get angry with them. In her attempt to understand the world, she asked a lot of questions of her teachers.

'They always got annoyed in the end when they couldn't explain. In hindsight, I've realised that some teachers didn't have the knowledge to answer.'

Today, Ida has friends she has chosen herself, who accept her for who she is.

'I'm not at all an unpleasant person — I have a very hard time being unpleasant. Everyone says I'm nice. I can make friends with new people in a shop, just like that.'

Ida used to love music and had a talent for the piano. She went to a music school, but had to quit playing when her rheumatism set in.

She has many creative interests, painting and drawing portraits of both people and animals, has three dogs, and likes to be out in nature.

Her childhood was lined with conflicts at home.

'I was a pain in the arse. There would be a fight as soon as anything didn't turn out the way I wanted. Mum and Dad would really have needed help and support as parents. Mum and I couldn't stand each other when I was still living at home.'

Both Ida and her mother wanted things their own way. Their relationship improved once Ida moved out.

'Later, when I started talking about going through the screening process, we realised that Mum has Asperger's, too! She went through life not knowing until she turned 60.'

With all the facts in hand, they can see clear signs of autism in Ida's grandfather as well.

Today, Ida and her mother are closer than ever and understand each other completely.

'It's like we can be "Aspies" together. I enjoy needlework, and Mum is so good at it. When the new embroidery catalogue comes out, we sit there and geek out together. It's rare having someone to share that kind of stuff with, being able to talk forever about something and laugh your arse off at things no one else gets. It's a good thing for my husband, too. When Mum and I are being Aspies, Dad and he can go grump a little in the sauna about how hard it is living with an autist — because it is. It's not always easy for them.'

She met her husband through a mutual friend when she was just 19 years old.

'It was like you only ever read about in books: love at first sight for us both. We just clicked right away. We dated for a month before moving in together.'

Ida and her husband wanted to live in a house, so they moved to the countryside and had two children. It took a long time for Ida to get used to the change. Her routines went away and day-to-day life got turned upside down. The big, new responsibility could overwhelm her. But today she feels secure in her role as a parent and finds it easy to know how the kids are doing or sense what they need. Children are honest. It makes them easier to read than adults.

'They show so clearly if they are angry or happy.'

But other everyday situations can be trickier. Ida tells me about a time when her young son was having a friend over and the kids were standing next to each other by the coffee table playing with toy cars. It got too crowded, and the boys started squabbling about space. Ida couldn't figure out how to solve the conflict. She sat down, trying to reason with her son, while the other boy's mother intervened and decided that one of the kids could walk around the table so that each had their own side. Immediately, the situation was defused.

'It wasn't harder than that. But I often get tunnel vision, and all I'm thinking is, "dear, oh dear, now they're fighting," and I don't see the simple solution.'

In the evenings, she experiences extreme mental fatigue, collapsing onto the couch, and has to take a break from all sound and movement. She needs a lot more rest than her husband. The most common preconception Ida encounters when telling others about her diagnosis is that she is too social to be autistic.

'And they assume that I'm really good at maths, which I'm terrible at. Others are surprised that I'm of normal intelligence, because they've got it into their heads that it means I'm less intelligent. Then you have to explain that we are all different as individuals, even though we share the same diagnosis.'

But the hardest thing to communicate, Ida says, has been her sensitivity to sensory input and the tiredness it brings. It's not easy for others to grasp that she can have the stamina to focus on her interests for long periods and at the same time feel exhausted after a single social commitment.

Ida tries not to push herself too hard to be the perfect mother.

'I don't have the energy to go do lots of activities with the kids as often as others. But they're no worse off for that — we do other things. One week, we put up new wallpaper in my daughter's room, and both the kids helped out. They thought it was fun and were just as tired as if we'd gone to a play centre.'

Ida involves the children in chores around the house because she wants them to be better prepared for adult life than she was. The kids help with folding laundry, baking, and rolling meatballs, and she fights the urge to intervene when the results are not perfect.

She doesn't shy away from asking family and friends for advice about situations she doesn't understand. And at every opportunity, she rests.

'Even though there are times when it's tough and difficult, I would never get by without my kids. I pat myself on the shoulder sometimes to remind myself that I'm raising them well.'

I explain to the psychologist in Hagsätra that I can't find my way anywhere and that my non-existent sense of direction is one of the things that has made me suspect I have autism.

I have no spatial awareness. Often, it feels as though the world is changing around me, but I'm standing still. It's like it has been turned inside out or I'm looking at it through a mirror. I walk up a hill and down the same way, but still end up in a different place than where I started.

My whole life, I have intuitively known that my inability to orient myself comes from inside me — that it has to do with something inside my own head. It can't be trained away. That it might have been caused by my environment growing up is unthinkable. As a child, I was allowed to roam freely on my own, yet I could never find my way.

In our family, it was said that I had inherited my mother's sense of direction. She always navigates by landmarks, mumbling methodically to herself 'taking a right by the shoe shop' in order to remember her way back — yet like me, she gets lost all the time. It took me several years after moving to Södermalm in Stockholm before I learnt to navigate the six or seven blocks from Medborgarplatsen to Mariatorget. When I called my husband to ask for directions, he thought I was messing with him. Then he gave me an explanation so vague that I got irritated. This same procedure was repeated about once a week.

At work, I have learnt which route to take to get to the studio, the lunch restaurant, or my office space. I can never try a new one; it always goes wrong. On occasion, I have tried to trick myself by walking in the exact opposite direction to the one that I think is right. Logically, I should end up in the right place if I deliberately go the wrong way. But it's hard to outsmart my legs when they want something. My body turns of its own accord — alas, always in the wrong direction.

My brain's so-called 'visuospatial functions', which are crucial when trying to orient oneself, are not cooperating. It's our visuospatial ability that allows us to discern shapes and outlines, distances, movement, and the way objects are placed in relation to each other.

Since the advent of GPS technology in mobile phones, I rarely get lost anymore. But my poor sense of direction shrinks my world. Not being able to orient oneself feels unsafe. It feeds an inner fear of the world, as every step outside the door is unpredictable. Nor do I recognise faces, so just to be safe I say hi to everyone.

When I was younger, the feeling could be intoxicating, as though the streets of the city lay open at my feet, each walk an adventure. Now that I'm a little older, I move with a mounting insecurity. My circles mustn't grow too big. For the same reason, I dislike travelling — other than to the Italian island I have visited every year since I was born. There is a sense of security in the old age of the houses and the culture. Italy doesn't change.

§

I walk the same route to work every day. I turn off at Stallgatan from Södra Blasieholmshamnen and walk towards Nybrokajen. When I pass Blasieholmstorg, the horse is right there on my left. Its front leg is raised as though in greeting, its skin a little creased by the front shoulder. I have always liked it.

On my way home, I usually take Arsenalsgatan up towards Kungsträdgården. At Blasieholmstorg, the horse appears again on my left as usual.

But one day I pause, turning my head and scanning along the walls of the buildings that line the square. That's when I see it. There is another, identical horse on the other side. There are two of them.

How many times have I walked here, along the streets on each side of the square — and yet I have always thought that the horse is one and the same. A frightening and familiar sensation of the surreal runs through me. I know that statues don't move. I know that. Why have I perceived reality as though it were possible? Or did I believe that I was walking down the same street, now a mirror image of itself? I begin to doubt my own faculties of perception. I'm unable to interpret the world. It frightens me. It appears unreliable and treacherously fickle.

Without knowing it, Sigmund Freud described the autist's anxiety and fear of the world better than anyone. He captures the feeling with great precision in his concept of *das Unheimliche* — the uncanny — which he introduced in a 1919 essay with the same title.

The uncanny is the feeling of unease that arises when the familiar is revealed to contain something alien. It can be a slight obliqueness, barely perceptible shifts that allow something unfamiliar to creep into an otherwise homely and safe environment. According to Freud, the feeling of the uncanny arises when we are faced with phenomena such as doppelgangers, deja vu, magic, epileptic seizures, and people speaking in tongues, when we are lost, or when we are unsure of whether something is a living creature or a dead object, human or machine.

Freud imagines that the uncanny emerges in the clash between a motif and certain long-lost ideas from the individual's deep past. The motif, such as the doppelganger, becomes a reminder of something long hidden; it triggers a repressed memory. Should that which has been brought to life have remained buried? To Freud, the uncanny marks 'the return of the repressed'.

A shift occurs. The world is warped. The crack in the sidewalk grows longer and deeper. The hidden, which should have stayed hidden, returns to the surface. During the past century, Freud's concept of the uncanny has been used to describe vastly different phenomena, from horror films to homelessness. His examples of what can be thought of as uncanny are many and diverse, which opens his text up to readings from multiple perspectives.

Yet the English translation of *das Unheimliche* as 'the uncanny' loses the connection in the German original to the word 'home', which specifies that the feeling arises in relation to the familiar. It's something homelike that changes character and becomes threatening. The German 'heimlich' can mean both familiar and homely as well as that which is safely secret and hidden.

This idea of the homely turned alien leads Swedish author Mara Lee to associate *das Unheimliche* with a horrific rationality and perverted correctness that believes itself to mean well but whose consequences are destructive. As when everything is done by the book and no one messes up, yet nevertheless the results are horrific. This gives a new resonance to those institutions of trust that are referred to as homes without being so: the day home, the retirement home, the care home. Places like Vidkärr Orphanage. Mara Lee refers to them as places to store people who don't have access to a home of their own. False homes in the name of equality, built for the purpose of levelling differences. Yet the ideal of this imagined community is conditional, requiring that everyone be the same. You have to be like us to be one of us.

To me, the uncanny is linked to the feeling of being a primitive individual, or remaining a child all my life. It's as though the child's fantasies and sense of reality never left me. Nothing is necessarily what it seems. The feeling of recognition is stolen from me, the rug beneath my feet disappears in one swift movement, and it all happens without warning.

In horror stories, the feeling of the uncanny is used to plant seeds and omens of greater disasters to come. In the author John Ajvide Lindqvist's short story collection *Let the Old Dreams Die*, one of the main characters builds a model ship out of matchsticks in his bedroom; when he gets up, he notices that the floor is sloping. Another character stands facing his teacher in front of the blackboard in the classroom and suddenly notices that the teacher has only one ear. A customs officer opens a bag, and among the clothes lies a larvae hatchery.

I run into a person in the street who seems familiar, yet I don't know who they are. I get lost in the corridors at work where I walk every day. I confuse two different mothers at preschool for the same person. Instead of the regular tree on the way to the bus stop, I see a person with their arms stretched out. The same bronze horse appears in different locations around the city where I live.

THE UNBEARABLE
WEIGHT OF BEING

Am I the only one who doesn't understand why people
scream at concerts?

QUESTION IN A FACEBOOK GROUP FOR

FEMALE AND NON-BINARY AUTISTS

'It's not very hard for autistic women to find a male romantic partner,'
says Svenny Kopp. This has become clear in her studies of autistic
women. 'The problem is finding a friend. A female friend.'

One prejudice about autists is that they suffer from a lack of
empathy. It springs out of the neurotypicals' expectations of mind
reading: they shouldn't have to give words to their problems; instead,
those surrounding them should grasp their problems intuitively. The
prejudice also grows out of an ignorance of the different forms of
empathy that exist.

Empathy researchers differentiate between cognitive and emotional
empathy, where autists may have a lack of cognitive empathy — that is,

they don't immediately understand how to react in a certain situation, what the different roles are, or what is expected of them. An outsider may mistake this for coldness.

But autists have no lack of emotional empathy — the ability to feel compassion, or affective empathy, which is to feel what the other person feels. On the contrary, autists feel very strongly for others, and many show great civil courage. Often, those feelings can become so overwhelming that the autist risks being completely consumed by the other person's emotions, making them her own.

When I was a child, it sometimes happened that others my own age became resentful without me understanding why. I realised that I must have been misunderstood somehow, but not when or how. A fear took root in me, and I began to minimise risks in my friendships by letting others decide, so that no one would get strangely annoyed like that. I often found myself in constellations that may have looked like a trio from the outside, but were really two best friends and one backup — me.

I listened, asked questions, said yes to every suggestion, expressed almost no needs of my own, kept confidences but rarely offered any in return, and became everyone's most amenable friend. I never knew when it was time to go home, so I always stayed last just to be safe.

When I grew older, I spent all my time at the stable. My relationship with horses felt peaceful and undemanding compared to that with other people.

But one of my friends continued to get inexplicably angry with me, for what I later understood were crimes against the conventions of girl friendship. In upper secondary school, she wanted us to talk for hours on the phone each night. I didn't get the point. I didn't know what to say, or why we had to repeat the same thing so many times. But I adjusted and learnt that a comment about a guy or a pair of jeans wasn't over and done with simply because we had said it once.

Later, I tried to find more of a sense of self, expressing more needs — but that didn't help, either. It didn't matter that I spoke without subtext and was being completely honest, I was still interpreted as though I meant something other than what I said.

It was easier to hang out with boys, especially those who were younger. Their communication was clearer. I was allowed to be childish and talk about my interests without constantly having to comply with the girls' complicated system of codes for social interaction. Girls were always looking outwards at the group and, in my eyes, were unreasonably fixated on what others thought of them. Everything in their world was emotionally charged and carried several layers of meaning. It was so easy to hurt them by accident, and it terrified me.

In my mind, I was fiercely loyal and willing to take big risks to defend those close to me. But I noticed that my idea of loyalty differed from theirs. I was rarely given a chance to show it, because they didn't expect the kind of fidelity I was capable of. Over the years, I began to see a pattern: I asked too much of my friends morally and was terribly disappointed when I realised that they weren't willing to sacrifice as much for me as I for them.

I didn't understand what was implied, couldn't decipher the codes. It was as though something went on between others — an invisible, silent force between them, something imperceptible, subtle, ever-changing. An exchange of meaning, a silent negotiation, a mutual understanding that arose so quickly it looked to me like telepathy.

In my 20s, I sought out a crowd that liked to party, and cultivated a tougher attitude. Around them, I didn't have to walk on eggshells. We went out more or less every night of the week. I loved chugging drinks and tumbling down from bar tops. Alcohol rendered ordinary social rules null and void. Everyone who was drunk acted strangely, and this was accepted. The clubs and the bars were safe zones, environments where I could behave any way I liked. Unexpected encounters and bizarre disputes turned into funny anecdotes as my friends and I constructed our mutual mythology.

Without knowing it, I was studying social interaction through the books, TV shows, plays, and films that I devoured. They were my study materials. I would often borrow lines and exchanges from them, not because I wanted to put on an act but because the words went straight into my mind and lodged themselves there, helping me understand some nuance better.

For me, cultural consumption was never an escape from reality. It was a way of getting closer to reality, of better understanding it, conquering it.

Some doubt the power of fiction to touch us to the core and influence our feelings and behaviours. They have never seen an autistic girl watch the same episode of a tween show on repeat, memorising each line so she can speak to her friends in the schoolyard.

I grew older, went to university, transformed my special interests into a profession — arts and culture journalist — and started working in radio and TV. There, communication was simpler; there were rules. For radio, you wrote a script before speaking and all you had to do was read it aloud. In peace and quiet, I could think about what I wanted to say, carving sharp little sentences into a text of two and a half minutes before reading it from the diaphragm with a voice that was filtered through the large compressor at Radio Sweden. No one was allowed to interrupt. 'Us who work here are the ones who weren't listened to as children,' a colleague at the culture desk once said to me. She cried often at work, and everyone agreed that she was the most brilliant among us. There was a colleague in the office who spoke fluent Chinese; rumour had it that another had partied with Ulrike Meinhof in Berlin. In the morning meetings, everyone directed merciless criticism at each other's segments.

In the studio, sound technicians who looked like woodwork-class teachers sat editing our speech on reel-to-reel tapes, often with cut-out strips of recording tape that needed to be added in somewhere strung around their necks. Pieces of tape with retakes and redundant words floated down to the floor. Sometimes an important 's' went missing and they had to dive down underneath the mixing desk to find it.

I loved reading out my radio scripts. When the green light came on in the studio, the floor was mine.

When my colleagues in the media precariat who were on temporary employment didn't get their contracts renewed — that is, had their jobs taken from them and were put in quarantine from the workplace because our employer didn't want to be forced to offer them a permanent job under the Employment Protection Act — I was furious and wanted to protest loudly and publicly. But few of them were even willing to admit that they had been treated poorly, and they didn't want to revolt. When it eventually became my turn to lose my job, few of my companions in misfortune in the temp trenches seemed to care, much less be upset. I felt betrayed, angry at what I perceived to be their cowardice, and amazed at people's ability to say things they didn't mean.

It took me a long time to grasp that those of us making radio and TV together in tight-knit but temporary teams were merely colleagues — not friends. It took me even longer to realise that we were also competing for jobs.

Social interaction pays no heed to the autist's compass, especially not in the media industry. You can't draw on your strengths if these conflict with the expectations of neurotypicals. Most conspicuous will be the aspects that are perceived as negative, like withdrawing, offering criticism that is too harsh, and avoiding big groups. Positive qualities like honesty are of little help in a world where a constant trickle of white lies is socially acceptable. Nor is loyalty useful in a context that expects a certain level of disloyalty.

The more high-functioning you are, the easier it is to study expected behaviours, mask your autism, and behave on the majority's terms — in social relationships, in the schoolyard, and on the job market. And the better you are at 'acting normal', the less seriously you will be taken when explaining your difficulties. Masking makes people depressed; it drains them of energy. It deprives them of the possibility of an authentic and true life.

My dreams about love were for a true equal. A best friend and confidant. I imagined that in a romantic relationship I would finally be free of all these fickle theatrics surrounding me — that the relationship could be a space where I was allowed to be fully myself.

By pure luck, I found my equal. We locked eyes one night at the student pub, did green shots, and danced close together. On the dance floor, he put his hand to his mouth in a sneeze. The phlegm stuck to his hand and he didn't know what to do, so he tucked it into his pocket, held me with his left arm, and continued dancing. I didn't notice a thing.

A few days later, we grabbed coffee and decided to be a couple. We were the same age and had the same opinions on everything. We played, laughed, made the same observations. We slept together under the skateboard ramp in Humlegården. He had a side job at the IT company Spray and pink business cards with a drawing of a giraffe and the title 'power surfer'. I moved into his sublet with a badly water-damaged bathroom, and we made up an imaginary creature that lived with us.

We belonged together with the same natural ease as a pair of siblings. I wore his clothes. We shared socks and had long conversations in distorted voices. We got drunk and talked about our parents. I forgot what my face looked like, because I only saw his. Our brains connected wirelessly from different sides of the room. We stayed together for 15 years and grew into adults in parallel. We became ourselves together.

We got married on my family's oft-visited Italian island when I was 28 years old. The wedding had been arranged by my parents. I don't know why we let them decide everything, but their ideas were dreamlike and grand. The wedding was organised as a presentation of the island to the 50 guests visiting from Sweden. Everything was admired: the landscape, the food, the people, our clothes. In the midst of all the ballyhoo, my husband and I stood there looking a little helplessly at each other. We were like two children together.

My mother had bought me a bridal dress for a small fortune and booked out a hotel where the wedding reception took place. The chef who cooked the food cut the meat standing on a podium in front of our applauding guests. The dinner was five courses, and that's after we had got rid of two.

My mother gave a speech painting me as someone politically engaged, and it was like she was talking about someone else. Dad was moving and ceremonious in his speech, saying that if things had been like in the past and the groom had to ask the bride's father for her hand, there was no one he would rather have knocking on his door than my husband.

We danced our wedding waltz on the terrace to 'Endless Love' by Diana Ross and Lionel Richie. The hotel owners opened the bar when they realised that the Swedes weren't going to settle for a small digestivo after dinner, preferring liquor mixed with soda in sizeable drinking glasses instead.

That night, we fell asleep exhausted in our hotel bed, still fully clothed. My dress had covered buttons down the back that we didn't manage to undo.

It was June of 2005. We were wed in the town hall by the city's mayor in an Italian civil ceremony. Someone took a photo of us that was pinned to the wall next to pictures of other couples — proof that we had lived and been there.

It was one of the happiest days of my life. But I only realised much later.

TOO MUCH FAITH
IN WORDS

Sometimes it feels like those of us with Asperger's or
autism are the only ones who can see through the noise.

GRETA THUNBERG IN THE FILM *I AM GRETA*

In September 2019, Greta Thunberg has been invited as a guest on
the American late-night talk and satirical news program *The Daily
Show* to speak about her commitment to the climate. The host, Trevor
Noah, mentions that her mother, the opera singer Malena Ernman, has
stopped flying — which means she is no longer able to go on tour to
faraway places.

'Do you sometimes feel bad that she can't perform, or are you more
excited that she's not part of, I guess, polluting the planet?' he asks.

'I don't care, honestly, about how she performs,' Thunberg says.

The audience laughs. Trevor Noah jumps, before flashing Thunberg a
big smile. They think that she is joking, intentionally expressing herself
with a cocky, careless attitude towards her mother. But Thunberg isn't

joking; she is simply answering the question.

Indeed, to her the climate is more important than whether her mother's international opera career suffers. It doesn't mean that she harbours ill intent or has it in for her mother.

In the Facebook group for female autists, members help each other interpret their neurotypical fellows. They write dejectedly about perpetual clashes and misunderstandings in encounters with other people. Often, it's about trivialities — little things that other people don't give much thought.

The author of one thread describes a scenario: 'If you're in the store and you've forgotten to grab a bag, sometimes the cashier will say: "Take one, and we'll sort it out next time." Does she actually mean that? Are you supposed to bring it up and pay for the bag next time you go grocery shopping? What if it's someone else at the till, then she'll never know I paid?'

The author of the thread asks her neurotypical partner, who complicates things even further by explaining that cashiers often say that when there are several people in line who might overhear the conversation, so as to uphold the rule about paying for carrier bags. If you are alone, on the other hand, you are often told: 'Don't worry about it, just take one.' Her partner also explains that paying for the bag next time is optional. 'If *I* were the cashier, I would EASILY remember who I'd told to take a bag on the condition that they pay next time,' writes the thread's author.

Another group member also mentions an incident at the grocery store. She was waiting in line to pay when another till opened next to hers and the line split in two. When she chose to stay where she was, she received a tap on the shoulder and was encouraged to switch to the newer, shorter line. But she didn't want to switch. She wanted to stay. The atmosphere grew awkward, as the other customers couldn't understand why she didn't want to switch to the shorter line. The norm is to always hurry, always be in a rush.

A third group member regretfully recalls forgetting her payment card at home and asking the cashier whether she could pay via an app that allows you to send money to other people's phones. The cashier had been offended and said no. 'Why was she so unkind?' the author of the thread wants to know. 'If it had been me, I would've said yes right away.'

'Of course you can't ask her that. She's at work and doesn't want to get her personal phone involved,' another group member comments.

'Okay, thanks for explaining,' comes the answer.

In the Facebook group, no one is offended by harsh words and blunt comments. Autists can express themselves drastically and let others do the same. The tone in the group is liberating; here are none of the maladies afflicting online debating among neurotypicals, like personal attacks, whataboutism, and straw men. People argue factually and stick to the subject.

The situations described in the Facebook group may seem mundane, almost meaningless, but seen together they paint a bigger picture. In our time, people are always expected to be in a hurry and it's thought of as normal to choose the fastest lane, the most efficient way of getting ahead. Promises to do the right thing about pocket change mean nothing; by unspoken agreement, they are merely polite conversation fillers that aren't meant to be realised.

'If they're such amazing communicators, you'd think they would be able to understand us,' a group member named J writes about neurotypicals. She has given up the thought of having a romantic relationship with a non-autist. She continues: 'No one cares about trying to teach the neurotypicals around us how to communicate with and listen to us. They are the ones who are supposed to have an intuitive natural talent for cognitive empathy and theory of mind and mind-reading, so you'd think it wouldn't be so damn hard.'

On the internet, there is also a community among autists who make fun of neurotypicals, painting them as the misfits. During the COVID-19 pandemic, they marvelled collectively at how much non-autists were complaining about having to stay home and take it easy. 'Caring for Your NT During Social Isolation' read a headline on the site neuroclastic.com.

For us, this is just another day of the week, the author pointed out, and ridiculed the neurotypical love of greetings. 'One of the most bemusing things that has come out of these recent weeks has been watching NTs bend themselves into bizarre contortions in order to touch each other in greeting without risking death to either party,' she writes. 'I can't understand why bumping elbows — the part of your body that you COUGH ON — is a good idea but there's a lot about NTs that I don't understand ... as if a simple hand wave isn't the first thing we teach babies. We also have words. They include hello, hi, good to see you, nice to meet you, and the perennial autistic favourite: simply launching straight into an interesting discussion without bothering with all that nonsense.'

The author of the article on neuroclastic.com felt a sense of schadenfreude watching neurotypicals fret about the future during the pandemic. 'They're feeling much the way autistic people feel most of the time ... We know how it feels to want something from the store but feel like you could die if you go out for it.'

The author offers tips to help neurotypicals: create routines while working from home; learn to enjoy quiet and stillness; use noise-cancelling headphones. 'Without the distractions of the outside world to occupy them, maybe they, too, will finally — FINALLY — learn the joys of small comforts.'

Autists use language to convey a message, not to make an impression. As an autist, opening your mouth to speak is like talking in a foreign language where you don't know the etiquette. Everything sounds curt and clumsy. You are like a tourist who desires nothing more than to blend in, but at the espresso bar all you can manage is: 'A coffee.' Period. Your language skills are not sufficient to couch the order in some elegant, friendly phrase. It is not your intention to be impolite — you simply can't find the right words for all the fluff around the message itself.

When the autist finds herself in a conflict, this is often what it's about. But misunderstandings just as often arise because non-autists read hidden meanings that aren't there into her words.

As a woman, I have come to understand that I'm expected to speak in code. That is what most people do. For this reason, I'm often interpreted as speaking with a subtext, even when there is none. In fights with my neurotypical ex-husband, he could claim that I actually meant something entirely other than what I had just said. It was confusing beyond words. My 'Oh, look at all this garbage!' meant just that; there was no hidden criticism like 'Why don't you ever take the trash out, you never do anything around here' between the lines. But that is what he heard. I, on the other hand, heard none of his hints, interpreting everything he said literally. Trying to decipher other people's subtext is a constant headache for autists.

I have a dear friend who is the most neurotypical person you could imagine. She moves through life with a savoir faire that is incredible to behold. Everyone likes her. She deals with conflict and gets her way without anyone feeling angry or hurt. For a time, I asked her to ghostwrite my text messages to my ex-husband — and suddenly he and I got along. For me, flattery and doctoring the truth felt like violating my own integrity. But it worked.

The word 'metaphor' is Greek and means 'to carry over' or 'across'. Metaphors transpose descriptions and scenes to a new context; they carry over in another direction. Two worlds collide. These worlds can be drastically different, but in an elegant, effective metaphor it is precisely this collision that clears the sky and broadens our senses.

Language borrows its eternal imagery from such motifs as roads, water, plants, games, and war. Linguists understand metaphorical language as a path that leads from a source concept to a target concept. The ability to interpret metaphors requires that you recognise the image that appears in your mind, and that you can relate to it. The image has to come together.

I sometimes struggle with metaphors because I get stuck translating the image into reality, no matter how established the metaphor is. My neurodivergent brain can't make the leap between the concrete and the abstract without stopping to brood over it.

I know it doesn't matter whether a metaphor is true or not, only that it is perceived as such. Nevertheless, I assess its truth value. For example, if someone says that they feel like they have been 'driving all day at 30 kilometres an hour', I can't help but wonder whether they mean this as something good or bad. Isn't it quite relaxing to be driving at 30 kilometres an hour? I realise that the metaphor probably means it has been a tedious and slow day. Then I feel secretly annoyed at the way we are all expected to prefer speed over slowness. At this point, quite a bit of time has passed and I have fallen behind in the conversation.

That's how it works when I, as an autist, get hung up on the details. I have to concretise before I can generalise. The downside is that conversations grind to a halt, I'm perceived as socially incompetent, and my brain begins to boil.

The power over the metaphor rests with the majority culture — the neurotypicals. In order for a metaphor to work, everyone must agree on its underlying values. We have collectively decided that the parts of a table that prop up the top look like human or animal legs. For this reason, we call them 'table legs'. Likewise, there is a consensus that an 'ass' is a foolish or stupid person, not someone who looks like a donkey.

Because I don't drive, take no interest in sports or war, and haven't done military service, I can't relate to car, sports, or war metaphors. I can grasp them on a purely intellectual level because I have learnt what they mean, but they aren't rooted in me. If someone says that life is like a roundabout, I understand that are talking about going round and round in a circle. But if you wanted to, couldn't you just take the first exit? And so, I keep brooding.

In his book *The Penny That Dropped*, the linguist Lars Melin writes that everyday metaphors are interpreted automatically. Within seconds, everyone listening has grasped what a metaphor means, even if they haven't heard it before. There is no need to translate the metaphor into reality. This spontaneity has been proven in numerous experiments. 'If the theory involving translation was accurate, it would take longer to process metaphors than plain language,' Melin argues. Well, it does — at least for me. I love plain language.

The values that govern the metaphors of our language, so-called 'conceptual metaphors', are relatively easy to spot and often the same across different cultures. Up is good and down is bad, because plants — our food and the basis for all life — grow upwards through the earth, and we imagine God up in heaven. That is why our spirits are high, we float on air, we feel like we are flying, and we have come up in the world. Upward movement comes with positive connotations.

What might an autistic metaphor look like? In a more autism-friendly world, expressions such as 'having many balls in the air' or being 'totally wired' would have strictly negative connotations, meaning that someone is close to a breakdown due to constantly having to shift focus.

Autists like to literalise symbols. As a child, the American researcher and autist Temple Grandin heard a priest talk about the door to the kingdom of heaven that exists before all people. Open it and be saved, the priest said. Grandin went searching all around the house and wasn't satisfied until she found a small wooden door leading out onto the roof. That must be it.

To make sense of a saying like 'a rolling stone gathers no moss', Grandin must first conjure in her head the image of the rolling stone on which no moss can gather, before she can figure out what it means.

But just because autists process sensory input differently, this doesn't mean they can't create metaphors of their own. On the contrary, a person with autism often inhabits a thought-world rich in metaphors and symbolism. But these are personal metaphors, not the metaphors of the majority. Autists often think metaphorically and associatively and experience objects like physical representations of — or symbols for — something else.

The autistic Australian author Donna Williams explains that she tends to compare new things that she encounters with things she is already familiar with. She recasts new objects into something familiar as a way of creating meaning and intelligibility for herself. A necklace with a black, shiny gemstone is a TV screen; a lift with tiled walls is a bathroom. She makes whatever associations she can based on what she already knows, and is constantly inventing new metaphors for herself.

For the retired professor Elisabet, the round virtual buttons on her smartphone turn into fried eggs because they have a circle in the middle. For a person who receives and processes information differently, metaphors become necessary to sort through and make sense of a neurotypical reality.

I, too, literalise images. I remember a surrealist art exhibition at Millesgården, just outside Stockholm, a few years ago. I walked around the room feeling a mounting irritation at the artworks being described as 'dreamlike' when they weren't dreamlike at all. Dreams don't look like surrealist paintings. Who has ever dreamt of a melting clock?

Another time, I was at a Cindy Sherman exhibition at Moderna Museet in Stockholm. In big, glossy photographs, she portrayed distorted versions of herself. In some, she was a cowboy; in others, a businesswoman. 'Theatres of the Self' read a headline from the curatorial statement. It was an exhibition about the creation of female identity through a kind of role play — the way we play-act in front of ourselves and others, and carry our identity like a mask.

I walked around the exhibition without understanding what the pictures were showing. They were supposed to portray the subconscious, but I saw no link between Sherman's staged selves and her — or all of our — insides.

This masquerade couldn't possibly be going in the subconscious, I thought. She is playing dress-up for the eyes of others. In the subconscious, we are all alone. There is no audience admiring our costume. There are no fake noses, no props lying around. The roles we play in front of ourselves are more complex than generic images of businesswomen laden with jewellery or cowboys on the plains. The self would see through these static, simplistic images. It's not so easily deceived.

I couldn't make the leap between the concrete and the abstract. For me, there was a conflict of meaning, and the enriching encounter that others seemed to experience didn't arise. Successful metaphors need to carry over from a source world to a target world in such a way that a sharp double exposure makes both worlds visible. But for me, what arises instead is often a paradox. The metaphor mystifies. It is my preoccupation with the details that gets in the way.

Certain older metaphors are more useful to me because they are concrete and thus clearer than their contemporary counterparts. I still ask 'is the tape rolling?' when recording for the radio, because a magnetic tape spinning inside a tape recorder is easier to grasp than a recording in a computer program. Most people do this. For example, we still 'go for a ride' even though we now travel by car rather than horse. Likewise, I'm looking forward to seeing my book 'typeset', despite the process being entirely digital and not involving lead type anymore. Old meanings disappear as society changes, but the words remain. We continue to call our writing tool a 'pen', without considering that the term originates from the Latin word for 'feather' and a time when people still wrote with a quill.

Like everyone else, I, too, tend to use metaphors without thinking about it. But sometimes my choice is affected. It feels wrong to say 'lots of new faces' when I mean that I have met lots of new people, because I don't relate to faces and have pitiful face memory. I prefer 'lots of new names' to describe the same situation.

There is a film genre about semantic misunderstandings that is particularly comforting to autists. It's the one where an outsider is unexpectedly thrown into a new, unfamiliar environment where they are received as a saviour. In the film *Being There* from 1979, Peter Sellers plays a gardener who manages to become appointed as an adviser to the president of the United States without talking about anything other than gardening. Everything he says about sowing and harvests, budding plants, strong roots, and the changes of the seasons is interpreted as metaphorical statements about the economy, crises, and the state of the market by the top politicians around him. All on their own, they translate his highly concrete words into abstractions and hold him up him as a new thinker.

The same thing happens in the comedy *Office Space* from 1999, about the triumph of a truth-teller. The main character, played by Ron Livingston, grows tired of his meaningless office job and speaks frankly and truthfully in front of two external consultants about how much time he wastes and how little he cares about his work. The more drastically literal he becomes, the more delighted are the consultants, who have been hired to investigate which employees lack motivation and should be fired. They draw the conclusion that he is bored because he is overqualified, and recommend that he be promoted to manager.

In the real world, truth-telling is one of the problems of social intercourse that affect people with autism.

§

With his book *The Empty Fortress* from 1967, the Freudian psychologist
Bruno Bettelheim was one of the first to liken the autistic condition to a
fort or a siege. He also compared autism to being held in a concentration
camp. The same year, Clara Claiborne Park's book *The Siege* was
published — with the subtitle: 'the battle for communication with an
autistic child'.

They both imagined autism as an impenetrable fort, where the autist
was locked up and couldn't get out. The idea was that there was a real,
true person living inside, behind the autistic wall. Bettelheim believed
that autism in children was caused by the parents' inability to bond
during important stages of the child's development and was a proponent
of the idea of 'refrigerator mothers'.

The metaphors pertaining to the image of a fort live on. Autism is
described in terms of battles and breakthroughs, attack and defence.
The idea that you could unpick the lock or break into an autistic child
to find and save the person inside recurs in the titles of some of the
American books published in the 21st century, such as *Between Their
World and Ours: breakthroughs with autistic children, Finding Ben: a
mother's journey through the maze of Asperger's*, and *Through the Glass
Wall: journeys into the closed-off worlds of the autistic*.

The presentation of autism as something alien and hidden inside a
human being, and the autist as a riddle to be solved, is also found in
photography. An advertisement for a treatment program at an American
centre that claims to be able to cure children with neuropsychiatric
disabilities shows an image of a child's eye looking through a keyhole.
The text below the image reads: 'We'll give you the keys to unlock their
world.'

Close-ups of faces and eyes are a recurring motif in the imagery
surrounding autism in advertising, journalism, and art. But in truth, such
images are not so much a metaphor for autism itself as they illustrate the
neurotypical's attempt to understand and solve its 'mystery'. These are
the images of a photographer encroaching on the autist with the camera

in search of the true, hidden individual inside — an image-maker who imagines that the eyes are the mirror of the soul and that the essence of autism can be captured by getting close enough. But there is nothing to see, of course. Autism is invisible. Instead, these close-ups perpetuate an antiquated view of differently abled people as belonging in an exhibit, put on this Earth for others to scrutinise and examine.

Images of children with autism can also illustrate a parent's grief and anxiety at feeling shut out. Often, these children are portrayed as lonely and isolated in a big, dangerous world, as in the American photographer Rosie Barnes's images of her neurodivergent son in the book *Understanding Stanley: looking through autism*, where the boy is often standing at a distance, facing away from the camera, alone in the shot. He is photographed together with toys, a swing, and a trampoline — all of which he does not use. The images express a loneliness, passivity, and absence. But whose is the loneliness? How Stanley feels, the observer will never know; we never see his face. He might be at peace with his own meaning-making in the present, altogether content ignoring the swing and the trampoline. It's the mother's own loneliness and feeling of disconnect that is expressed in the images, not her son's.

The psychologist Jac den Houting, herself an autist, stands barefoot on a stage, saying that we have to redefine our understanding of autism. The medical sciences have taught us that there is a right and a wrong way for our brains to develop. Autism is consistently described in terms of *deficits* — it causes difficulties and problems. But den Houting felt liberated when she received her diagnosis.

'How could something that was so positive for me be such a bad thing?' she asks rhetorically in her TED talk.

When den Houting kept digging, she found other definitions of autism, formulated by people who were autists themselves. According to them, autism was part of the range of natural variation in human neurological development. They simply saw autism as a different way of thinking and emphasised that no brain is right or wrong. All forms of neurological development are equally valid and equally valuable.

But many people tend to compare autists, says den Houting. As a high-functioning autist, she is often put in contrast to someone who — according to the neurotypical layman's assessment — is 'really autistic'. Not just a little different, but truly 'disabled'.

'Maybe you can't tell just by looking at me, but I'm disabled, too. I'm not disabled by my autism, though. I'm disabled by my environment.'

The prevailing view on disabilities is called the 'medical model'. According to this model, disability is an individual problem, located within the disabled individual. Den Houting takes herself as an example.

'I really struggle with shopping malls. They're loud, they're brightly lit, they're unpredictable, they're full of people. The medical model would say that I struggle with shopping malls because there's a problem with the way my brain processes that input — because I'm autistic.'

But if there were shopping malls that were quiet, dimly lit, predictable, and sparsely populated, den Houting's difficulties would cease. Her abilities would no longer be 'impaired' by the shopping mall. Yet she would still be autistic.

Her point is that society *makes us* disabled. A disability arises when society counteracts, or clashes with, a person's individual characteristics.

Move to the countryside then, some might say. But wouldn't it be a shame if part of the population had to flee the cities and other people, simply to bear life on this planet?

Den Houting wants to use the word *disabled* not as a noun, but a verb.

'Disability is something that is being done to me. I am actively being dis-abled by the society around me. When I go to a shopping mall, I don't struggle because there is something wrong with me. I struggle because the shopping mall is designed in a way that doesn't cater to my needs.'

In den Houting's home country, Australia, the medical model dominates the understanding of autism, she says.

Globally, hundreds of millions of dollars are spent on autism research annually. The assumption is that autism is a problem to be solved. When den Houting looked at the allocation of research funding over the past ten years in Australia, she discovered that more than 40 per cent had gone to genetic and biological research, partly into the causes of autism, partly to find out whether it could be prevented. Another 20 per cent went to research into treatments for autism — how to make autists stop behaving autistically and start fitting in better with the rest of society. Only 7 per cent of funding went to research into helping and making life easier for autists.

Den Houting belongs to a younger generation of autists who are agitating online and on social media for their right to live an authentic autistic life. Drawing inspiration from identity-politics movements, they take pride in their diagnosis and demand respect and understanding. They want to reclaim the language to describe autism, arguing that neurotypicals are not best suited to speak about autism as they can't relate to the autistic experience.

It is this new generation of activists who are critical of the terms 'high-functioning' and 'low-functioning'. Who really has the right to call someone else 'low-functioning' simply because they function differently? What does it matter if a person doesn't speak or write like the majority? We are all equal as autists, these activists argue on social media.

Svenny Kopp doesn't agree. Because the autism spectrum is so wide, we need terms to differentiate between people. The difference between a person who works full-time in a demanding job and someone who can't speak or hear is vast. If we refer to both of them simply as 'autists', the one with the most obvious traits will come to define what autism is.

Once again, high-functioning women risk becoming invisible.

'We have to be able to differentiate based on the need for support, but not so as to degrade or stigmatise,' she says.

Kopp still receives regular letters from desperate parents of autistic girls and young women who write that they aren't taken seriously or getting the right help. They aren't believed at school because the girls are quiet and do well on their schoolwork.

She is currently conducting a follow-up study of the girls she worked with in the 1990s, who are now around the age of 35. Her groundbreaking research and refusal to give up has been the salvation for many autistic women.

One of them is the author Lina Liman, whose aunt just happened to hear Kopp speak about autism in girls on the radio and recognised her niece's symptoms. By then, Liman — severely anorexic and depressed — had spent seven years in psychiatric inpatient care and almost lost her life. None of the many doctors and psychologists she had met had figured out that she was autistic. But the radio interview set her on the right track, and by the age of 32 she had finally received her diagnosis. In *The Art of Faking Arabic*, she writes that Kopp's research gave back her life.

THE AUTISTIC BRAIN

But you have a life. I have a routine.

CYNTHIA NIXON IN THE ROLE OF EMILY DICKINSON

IN THE FILM *A QUIET PASSION*

Temple Grandin has an asymmetrical brain. On the MRI scans, you can see that one ventricle — a fluid-filled cavity in the brain — on the left is almost twice the length of the ventricle on the right. The sac-like bladder is so long that it extends into the parietal lobe, the part of the brain that houses our working memory.

How did this difference arise in Grandin's brain?

Grandin was born in Boston in 1947, three years after Hans Asperger had published his initial research findings. Almost no one knew what autism was.

As a three-year-old, Grandin showed no signs of beginning to speak. She would throw tantrums and often disappeared into her own world. Her mother brought her to a neurologist, who did an EEG to check whether the girl had epilepsy and carried out a hearing test to rule out deafness.

'She's an odd little girl, but she'll learn how to talk,' the doctor concluded. Then he classed Grandin's odd behaviour as a brain injury and referred her to a speech therapist.

If Grandin had been born just a decade later, she believes, the assessment would have been different. Then, her mother would probably have been told that her daughter was mentally ill and that she should send the child off to an institution. Her mother would herself have been viewed as a 'refrigerator mother' — one of those who were 'just happening to defrost enough to produce a child', as Leo Kanner said in *Time* magazine in 1960.

But in 1947, it was too early for all that. Grandin's doctor merely noted that there was something wrong with the girl's brain; he didn't have any treatment suggestions. Her mother didn't have to carry the blame for failing as a parent and was left to focus on helping her daughter in peace. She accepted that she was powerless over the cause but understood instinctively what her daughter needed. Grandin's mother constructed her own social-interaction exercises and practised with her daughter for several hours each day. Many of her self-invented methods were similar to those that would be recommended by behavioural therapists decades later, Grandin notes in her autobiography. Her mother was before her time.

Today, the 75-year-old Grandin is one of the most famous autism experts in the US. She has given innumerable lectures and written books about her autism that have sold more than a million copies. There is an Emmy Award–winning HBO film about her life with Claire Danes in the leading role.

Grandin's brain has been scanned eight times. The exams show that her brain is 15 per cent bigger than average; she has more white matter in her left hemisphere than do people in the control group; and her amygdala is larger, which is common in autists. The scans also show that her cerebellum — the part of the brain in charge of motor skills, posture, and balance — is 20 per cent smaller.

Today, scientists agree that autism is found in the brain. There is an incontestable connection between autistic behaviour and the functions of the brain. But the spectrum is wide, and autistic brains don't all look the same.

For Grandin, the neurologists' conclusions confirmed what she had long sensed. She has always had an exceptional visual memory. It has felt as though she is 'over-connected' in the brain and has a 'direct line' to the visual cortex, which facilitates visual memory. MRI scans of her brain have shown that her metaphor describes a concrete reality: her brain truly is 'over-connected'.

Inside the cerebral cortex is the white matter containing bundles of nerve fibres that facilitate communication between neurons. The fibres form neural pathways. In the images of Grandin's brain, two so-called 'subcortical pathways' stand out from the rest. Among other things, these pathways connect different parts of the brain and transmit processed visual information to the frontal lobe. Grandin has more connections than the standard brain, and the scans show thick pathways with one bundle of fibres extending all the way to the visual cortex.

Despite her mother doing everything she could to teach her daughter about social interaction, Grandin had a troubled childhood. She found it difficult to connect with the people around her, but felt a greater affinity with animals. They required no intricate social codes. Her love of animals led her to become one of the world's foremost experts on livestock.

In the US, attitudes towards autism have changed significantly in recent years, much thanks to Grandin's awareness-raising efforts. In shaping public opinion, she has increased understanding and highlighted positive aspects. To her, it's clear that autism can be an asset to the individual, if only they are given the right conditions. She also believes that autism should be understood symptom by symptom, not as some catch-all umbrella diagnosis. For instance, she divides autistic thinking into three different specialised categories: visual thinking, pattern thinking, and verbal/logical thinking. With this division, she wants to help autists identify their strong suits. Grandin herself is a visual thinker. Her extraordinary visual memory has helped her construct intricate solutions for keeping livestock. She has invented complicated new systems of ramps, handling chutes, and corrals simply by visualising them.

But interacting with people has been more difficult. To the neurologist Oliver Sacks, she described her life as being 'an anthropologist from Mars' — a researcher constantly looking for signs of intelligibility in a strange universe. With herself as the object of study in countless books, lectures, and articles, she has had an immense significance for the growing knowledge about autistic people.

Grandin is a pragmatic and stubborn person who finds her own solutions to her problems. When she identified a bodily need to be touched, she constructed a 'squeeze machine' — that is, a remote-controlled hug machine that she can lie down in. She doesn't want other people to touch her, but the squeeze machine has a soothing effect as it envelops her entire body and exerts a gentle pressure on it. The inspiration came from the narrow cattle crushes and treatment boxes used to keep livestock still during branding or veterinary exams.

At Grandin's high school, there was a teacher who noticed her interest in machinery and livestock keeping and took it seriously. He encouraged her to learn to construct and build on her own. In the clarity of scientific language, she found liberation from the unspoken assumptions and undefined feelings that characterise social language. She had found her place.

In the beginning of her career, it happened that she was tricked and exploited because of her difficulty interpreting and seeing through body language. At one of the cattle ranches Grandin had designed, the machinery would often break. No one understood why. After repeated incidents, she noticed that it only happened when a certain man named

John was in the room. She drew a connection between his presence and the broken equipment and realised that he was sabotaging the facility. Grandin learnt cognitively to be suspicious — she could put two and two together but hadn't seen the jealousy in John's face. For some men in the livestock industry, it was difficult to accept that a female autist could so easily construct the equipment that they needed.

Today, Grandin is a professor at Colorado State University. She has lived for her work and never had a romantic relationship.

Scientists have sought to answer these questions: What does an autistic brain look like? And what does it do differently compared to a neurotypical brain? Many answers have been found, but we still have far to go before we can diagnose autism simply through brain imaging.

The causes of autism are biological and mainly hereditary. But how does an autistic brain turn out the way it does? Why do these abnormalities arise?

The answer is that it involves many genes. And many of these many genes have a role to play in the growing brain, especially in the formation of neurons and communication between brain cells. Here we see minor variations in the genetic code controlling the brain's development. But the variations don't look the same in everyone. A genetic variation that is found in one autistic child might be absent in another. Autism is not like Down syndrome, for example, which we have long known is caused by an extra copy of chromosome 21.

Autism is a wide umbrella diagnosis that expresses itself through traits that may be shared but not identical in every person. In recent years, scientists have come to understand that many different gene mutations and genetic variations are required to create even a single autistic trait in an individual. The combination that gets inherited is crucial.

§

In people with autism, scientists have observed a significantly higher blood flow in several parts of the brain compared to neurotypicals. One such area with a more active blood flow is the cerebellum.

If you were to make an incision straight through the cerebellum, you would see the grey cerebral cortex and the brain's white matter form a branch-like pattern. The cross-section cuts through the cerebellar vermis, the cerebellum's mid-section, with its thin transversal lines. This grey-and-white pattern is known as 'arbor vitae', or 'the tree of life'.

I study a picture of the cerebellum. The delicate white branches of the brain matter in the tree of life remind me of a medieval church mural where the foliage has faded due to lime-washing and restorations. In biblical legend, the Tree of Life is bare, with no bark or flowers. It cannot grow for the sins of Adam and Eve.

The Tree of Life is often represented as three trees grown into one — cedar, olive, and spruce or cypress. In one story, an aged Adam sends his son Seth to the gates of Paradise to retrieve a branch from the Tree of Life. By the cherub with the flaming sword, Seth is given three seeds to place under his father's tongue once he is dead. When Adam dies, he is buried on Mount Zion, and from his grave three shoots spring up. David finds them and brings them to the Kidron Valley, where they grow together into one single enormous tree. Centuries go by, and when Christ is about to be crucified, a cross is needed. The old trunk is harvested and the timbermen discover that it consists of three trunks grown into one. From the cedar, they make the vertical post; from the cypress, they make the crossbeam; and out of the olive, they fashion the wooden plate where Pontius Pilate's inscription will be carved. Then, the cross is erected on Mount Zion. When Jesus is crucified, a stream of blood pours from his wounds and down along the cross. The blood trickles deeper into the earth and, like an oil of mercy, it cleanses Adam's skull where he lies buried. The head of humanity's sinful father is anointed with the oil of mercy from Paradise. And so, the story comes full circle.

According to neurology, I have an unusual amount of blood coursing around the tree of life in my cerebellum. The legend has found its way into my head, and I like the thought of the blood flow as an oil of mercy, in there among the branches and the grey folds.

Early descriptions of the brain imagined a landscape of trees, animals, and islands. One area is known as the 'insula', from the Latin word for 'island', and is the part of brain that receives information about our inner and outer worlds. It receives all the signals from the body — how fast our heart is beating, how high our blood pressure is, and the way we are breathing — but it also receives information from our senses. On the island of the brain, our inner and outer worlds converge, and from this synthesis our brains create feelings.

The American poet Emily Dickinson lived in the 19th century, during a time when autism did not exist as a diagnosis. Yet she knew that she was different. Several of her nearly 1,800 poems are about her brain. In them, she describes it as splintered, swaying and swerving, a mind abandoning well-trodden routes for new paths, following its own currents, flooding and trampling down.

In poem 867, she writes that it feels as though her brain has been cleft in two. She tries to stitch it back together but fails. Her consciousness is in pieces, and the pieces don't fit together. She tries to link up her thoughts, join the past to the present, but sounds and language come undone, and the sentences elude her like balls she has dropped — or perhaps like balls of yarn, rolling away across the floor.

The psychiatrist Lorna Wing has described this experience of fragmentation as the autistic consciousness struggling with central coherence — that is, piecing together information from the past and the present, making sense of experiences and learning from them, understanding what will happen in the future, and making plans. The autist struggles to find her place in time and space and to create a totality out of details.

In poem 340, Emily Dickinson describes a funeral in her brain as well as dark thoughts where she is repeatedly tormented by drumbeats, treading boots, and bells tolling. A breakdown has taken place.

But Dickinson is also stubbornly proud of her peculiar mind. In poem 598, she writes that her brain is wider than the sky and deeper than the sea. And in poem 620, she insists that 'Much Madness is divinest Sense'.

How are we to understand autism as a phenomenon? The medical model tells us that autism is something one 'has' and should be treated. Then, there is the so-called 'neurodiversity model', which defines autism as an extreme variation within the range of the 'natural', something that can be expected. Some people grow to be seven foot six, which is rare but not a disease. They will, however, struggle to function — because society is not built for them.

The two models don't negate each other. Autism can at the same time be considered natural and be linked to other diagnoses and diseases. Genes for autism overlap with ADHD, dyslexia, and epilepsy. Close to 75 per cent of all children with autism have some other diagnosis, too.

Gene variants come about as DNA segments are switched out or fall away during the course of evolution. Genetic variation is the reason we are of different height and have different eye and hair colour. Some gene variants can increase the likelihood of certain diseases or conditions, while others can act as a protection. Both common and rare gene variants contribute to the likelihood that a person will develop autism.

New gene mutations can arise spontaneously due to 'environmental factors'. Such factors may include the mother or father's age, medications, environmental toxins, illness during pregnancy, or complications at birth. In other words, these environmental factors don't refer to the environment in which the child grows up, but to the way genes may be affected during pregnancy and birth.

Estimates of how much is hereditary and how much is down to environmental factors show that the heritability is about 80 per cent. This means that up to 80 per cent of autistic behaviour can be explained by inherited genes, and 20 per cent by environmental factors. Thus, environmental factors play a significantly smaller role than heredity.

This is not only true for autism. There are 80,000 man-made chemical substances. It would be impossible to test them all. But research has shown that older parents have an increased risk of gene mutations — the same is true in, for example, Down syndrome — and that an infection during pregnancy doubles the risk of autism. The latter has to do with the response by the immune system, not the virus itself: the fetus can be damaged by a strong immune response, by how intensely the body fights to get rid of the virus. It's also known that anti-epileptic drugs such as valproate can affect the fetus, as well as a low body weight in the mother, or excessive alcohol consumption.

One Swedish study of mothers who had fled to Sweden during their pregnancy showed an increased risk of the children developing autism or an intellectual disability. The study speaks of 'migration stress' activating the stress response system, which in turn affects the fetal environment.

Other environmental factors that have been discussed include vitamin-D deficiency, malnutrition, and extreme preterm birth, which we know can affect the brain's development. In a study from the Karolinska Institute, 22 per cent of premature babies showed signs of autism at the age of five. The proportion of people with autism is somewhat higher in Asia — why, we don't know. Children of Somali parents in Stockholm and Gothenburg also have a higher prevalence of autism, without scientists being sure why.

You can't tell from looking at a brain whether it is autistic, and the knowledge of what brain imaging can show is still limited. Sven Bölte, professor of child and adolescent psychiatric science at the Karolinska Institute, doesn't believe that the science will reach a point where it is possible to diagnose autism through brain scanning during his lifetime.

§

During a visit to the halls of the Apostolic Palace, the official residence of the pope in Vatican City, the psychiatrist Irina Manouilenko caught sight of a big toe. The toe was attached to a foot belonging to a man depicted in a mural on the wall.

More than anything, it was the space between the big toe and the rest that caught her attention.

The fresco *Disputation of the Holy Sacrament* is found in a room that used to be the pope's private library and was completed in the year 1510 by the Renaissance artist Raphael. It depicts the triumph of the church. Near the lower edge of the mural, on Earth among the people, a discussion is raging about the great mystery of the Holy Communion, involving among others the writer Dante Alighieri and the Dominican friar Girolamo Savonarola.

On the marble steps next to St Augustine sits a young man writing; he is taking dictation from the church father. From underneath his robes, a bare foot peeks out. The space between the big toe and the rest is conspicuous.

Manouilenko, who was in the middle of working on her doctoral thesis on the biological causes of autism, jumped at the sight of the foot. A wide space between the big toe and the rest is a so-called 'minor physical anomaly' that can occur in people with autism and other genetic syndromes.

In the research, there is a hypothesis that such minor physical anomalies are linked to spontaneous gene mutations during the fetal stage that affects the development of the brain. Such minor anomalies occur in people without autism, too, but a study that Manouilenko and her colleagues have conducted shows that they are more common in autists.

It is possible that sitting on the wall of the pope's former library — where the most important documents of the Catholic Church were signed — is a 500-year-old autist.

§

Changes in our genetic make-up may leave an impression on the development of the brain and the way we turn out. This can lead to an abnormality in, for example, our cognitive or intellectual abilities: thinking, planning, and organising based on a goal-oriented behaviour.

Via neuropsychology, we know that certain areas of the brain are of significance to certain functions. In the temporal lobe, for instance, there is an area that has to do with social functioning, and the so-called 'parietal' parts of the brain are involved in making sense of metaphors and implicit meaning. Difficulties with coordination and motor skills have been linked to abnormalities in the cerebellum.

Irina Manouilenko explains how brain imaging works to collect information about brain activity on a local level. It's possible to differentiate between blood that is rich or poor in oxygen and study changes in the brain. Often, the person being examined is placed in an MRI machine and given a task related to social functioning so that researchers can observe the activity in the brain. But in her doctoral thesis, Manouilenko used a PET scan — positron-emission tomography — to measure blood flow in the brain at rest — that is, when the research subjects weren't carrying out a task.

The results showed a marked increase in blood flow in several regions in the right side of the brain in individuals with autism compared to the control group. Autists have an increased blood flow to the cerebellum and parts of the cerebral cortex compared to neurotypicals. This means an increased activity — that is, a higher energy consumption — in the brain cells. The autistic brain is quite literally working harder.

When the Hollywood star Daryl Hannah walks the red carpet at a film premiere, she pretends that she is the hostess of the party; that she, and not the production company, is the one who has invited all the media and fans; and that it's her task to make the guests comfortable. It helps her deal with the high-pressure situation, which involves dazzling spotlights, a rapid pace, and shouting photographers. In her glory days, she often wore sunglasses to premieres.

Hannah was diagnosed with 'borderline' autism in the 1970s. The doctors wanted to send her off to an institution, but her mother refused and moved with her daughter from Chicago to Jamaica, in the belief that a change of scenery would do her daughter good.

As a child, Hannah couldn't sleep at night. She lay awake watching films instead. She was shy and socially awkward. In school, she got bullied.

At the age of 11, she decided to become an actress — not because the work itself felt alluring, but because she wanted to transport herself physically to the magical places she had seen in the movies, like the land of Oz in *The Wizard of Oz*. She longed for these strange worlds, for places where she could be herself.

There is a pattern in the roles she has chosen throughout her career. Often, she has played an outsider, an odd figure who ends up in a world where she is alone in her strangeness. She has been a half-fish out of water, a lone Cro-Magnon woman among Neanderthals, and a robot in the world of humans. She has been drawn to science fiction and films that interrogate what it means to be human; she has found herself in the borderlands between human and machine or human and animal. Her roles have had few lines, relying instead on modes of communication beyond spoken language. She is a non-speaking mermaid in *Splash*, a taciturn replicant in *Blade Runner*, a one-eyed assassin out for revenge in *Kill Bill*, a sexy giant in *Attack of the 50 Foot Woman*, and a Stone Age outcast in *The Clan of the Cave Bear*.

But her finest performance is in a role that seems likely to lie close to her own personality — as the shy, awkward hairdresser Annelle in the drama *Steel Magnolias*. Annelle is so uncomfortable in her own skin that in every shot she looks like she is about to crawl right out of it.

§

Films that profess to portray autism are a sad chapter in Hollywood history. Autistic characters are rarely portrayed in their own right. Instead, they are used as a curiosity in order to teach the neurotypical main character valuable life lessons. The neurodivergent presence becomes a plot device — an obstacle that must be conquered and which facilitates the development of the other characters.

The most famous example is Dustin Hoffman's autistic character Raymond in *Rain Man*. He teaches his emotionally stunted brother, Charlie, to become more empathetic. Raymond is also a savant — a popular stereotype about autists.

In older films, autism is portrayed as something that can be cured. Here, the condition turns into a challenge to overcome for the family surrounding the autist. In the film *House of Cards* from 1993, the girl Sally's autism goes away when her mother starts showing her love, and the family becomes whole again.

Autism has also been used as a tool to create tension in thrillers like *Silent Fall* from 1994, in which an autistic boy who does not speak witnesses his parents' murder. The boy is portrayed as locked inside himself, held captive by his condition. In one scene, the camera focuses on his expressionless face, zooming in on his eyes. A therapist who has been called in asks: 'What are you seeing in there?' The child is the keeper of a secret that his autism prevents him from disclosing. Even though the boy appears to be at the centre of the film, the real story is that of the therapists' diverging views on his treatment.

Later in the film, the boy is freed from his autism and begins to speak. One of the therapists concludes that autism is in fact a paralysing fear of the world. 'There is a boy in here. I just think he's trapped behind a wall. And I think the fact that he's trapped makes him terrified,' he speculates. Truth, light, and justice are all linked to the boy being 'freed' from his condition.

The film *Snow Cake* from 2006 tells the story of a female autist played by Sigourney Weaver. Her character, Linda, is literal, bound by strict routines, and hypersensitive to sensory input. But the true main character of the film is Alex, played by Alan Rickman. Linda's odd behaviour challenges Alex, making him re-evaluate and change his life.

The inability to portray neurodivergent characters as whole human beings lives on into our own decade, but the demands for representation in motion pictures have changed. The singer-songwriter Sia received harsh criticism for casting a non-autistic actor in an autistic role in her film *Music*, and for having the autistic character function as moral inspiration for the drug-dealing main character, Zu.

Two films about autistic women stand out as a cut above the rest. One is the HBO production starring Claire Danes as Temple Grandin. The other is Terence Davies' biographical drama *A Quiet Passion*, about the poet Emily Dickinson, who is played by Cynthia Nixon with a mix of rigidness and naivety.

In one of the key scenes in the film, the poet speaks in confidence with her sister-in-law, who expresses her admiration of Emily's writing and uncompromising attitude to life.

'But you have a life. I have a routine. It is God's one concession to a no-hoper,' Emily replies. 'Rigour is no substitute for happiness.'

In another scene, she stands dressed all in white at the top of a staircase, scolding her editor for changing the punctuation in her poems. Later in the film, she is shown falling ill with seizures and kidney disease, which takes her life at the age of 55.

What would be a true autistic narrative? In Andy Warhol's 1964 film *Empire*, the camera rests without interruption on the Empire State Building for more than eight hours. Perhaps this is the only truly autistic film in the world.

Another candidate is the five-minute-long, silent opening sequence of the sun rising over the sea at Sandhammaren, at the southernmost tip of Sweden, in Stefan Jarl's documentary *Time Has No Name*. Written on a sign is a Pier Paolo Pasolini quote: 'There is no poetry other than real action.'

The hardest thing about high-functioning autism is that you are too 'normal' for your difficulties to be taken seriously, but also too different to fit in. My feeling is that others possess an intuitive knowledge that I lack. It's as though they were psychic: they know how to respond, how to interpret and decipher; they have a map and a pre-existing understanding with which they have simply been endowed. I have studied and learnt a lot — many would probably perceive me as socially gifted. But they cannot see the effort I put in and the price I pay in terms of exhaustion afterwards.

Autistic women are good at masking their social shortcomings because from a young age girls tend to be drilled harder in social intercourse than boys, both by the adult world and in their friendships. To mask my social inability as an adult, I have developed a strategy to step into my professional role as a journalist. When I find myself in a social situation with people I have never met before, I start to interview them. I ask questions, which most people appreciate, as it makes them feel seen.

The reason that women's autism is different from men's is partly that society places different expectations on girls and boys. Girls with autism learn early to hide their social difficulties. But their alienation also runs deeper, as women more so than men are expected to be socially driven and take responsibility for the wellbeing of others. Many autistic traits aren't compatible with women's traditional roles. Among these traits: not enjoying talk about feelings and relationships, preferring to sit alone in one's room and immerse oneself in one's own interests, having a hard time grasping subtext, and not being able to sugar-coat one's words.

Masking happens unconsciously. It starts at an early age as the child studies and mimics the play and speech of their peers. Children with autism tend to withdraw and make themselves invisible, as they carefully observe their fellows before attempting to copy them. Girls with autism are often interpreted as 'sweet', shy, and acquiescent. They don't take up space in a group or stir up trouble. By adulthood, their masking can be so honed that they become good actresses and social chameleons who blend in seamlessly in any company. By then, the long-term suppression of their own true self has often led to exhaustion and depression.

It is easy to imagine the alienation of autistic women throughout history, as women have carried the main responsibility for the home — that is, exactly the kind of practical chores that autists often struggle with. Sitting down and immersing oneself in a narrow special interest has been a privilege reserved for men. If women have historically cared for atypical men and been responsible for the social aspects of family life, then who took care of the odd women?

Yet Svenny Kopp thinks that it's harder to be an autistic woman today than in the past. She believes that the era of the housewife in the first half of the 20th century was one of the quieter historical periods for autistic women, as they could stay in the home and were provided for financially. Housewives in the cities could live rather sheltered lives, assuming that they had a good husband or stood under the protection of other family members.

'Our time, on the other hand, is challenging and incredibly difficult,' says Kopp. 'It's stressful, everything happens very fast, you're expected to be social. The demands are greater, and school has become less structured ... Women are expected to succeed in all areas. You're supposed to have kids, look good, have a good job. Doing all of this isn't possible. It's too hard.'

As early as in the 1920s, the British psychoanalyst Joan Riviere wrote about 'womanliness as a masquerade'. In her time, it was intellectual women wearing their feminine identity as a mask that could be put on when the need arose. By acting 'womanly' according to the norms of the time, they toned down their intelligence and acted less capable. It was a way of manoeuvring and surviving in the patriarchy. Their masking also turned into a method for avoiding anxiety about being different.

A person wearing a mask can be interpreted as someone who is concealing and pretending, deceitfully misleading those around them. The masque is something that dims the world; it represents falseness, appearance, and pretence.

Yet the autistic woman is not masking with the intention of being deceitful. Her true self is invisible even to her own person. She is masking to fit in, and doing so unconsciously. Often, she doesn't even understand that she has been camouflaging herself until she gets her diagnosis. Before that, she thinks her struggle is everyone else's, too. At least, that's what it was like for me.

As a high-functioning autist, you relate to the rest of the world as though it were an object of study. You observe, register, draw conclusions, commit to memory, and mimic. You become an imitator, in some cases even an expert on body language and interpersonal relationships. Every time I meet someone, I remind myself to look the other person in the eye. My impulse is always to turn down my gaze, since I experience eye contact as intimate and intrusive. I think better if I'm allowed to look away when I speak. The effort it takes to maintain eye contact is the same every time, even though I have practised all my life.

When people speak of the autist's strong suits, they usually emphasise things like the ability to think differently and the courage to call out injustice. Having a truth-teller in the group can, for instance, be much needed in the workplace.

But there is one catch. Just because something is good for the group, it doesn't necessarily mean that it's good for the individual. Always standing out wears away at the soul. Being different is draining, and so are the attempts to adapt, as they involve precisely that: adapting the self — being inauthentic.

Anxiety is the feeling of not being in harmony with oneself, wrote the philosopher Søren Kierkegaard. As a masking autist, you are constantly out of harmony with yourself. And moving through a neurotypical world without masking at all is near impossible for an autist. There would be too many conflicts and misunderstandings, as neurotypical people have a hard time grasping that not everyone is like them.

There is a social-media movement — primarily in the English-speaking world — that is all about making autism part of one's identity and highlighting its positive aspects. With hashtags like #aspiegirl, #aspielife, and #autisticpride, users exchange experiences, write about their everyday life, and post funny memes. There are lists of the perks of being an autist and lists of the strange things that neurotypicals do. In Facebook groups and on Instagram, the usual perspective is inverted, turning autism into the norm and neurotypicals into outliers. There, autists share tricks and strategies and support those who aren't doing so well.

This positive view of autism is part of a wider identity-politics movement that has swept across the world in the past decade, in which minorities are demanding a renegotiation of the social norms that have previously left them invisible or oppressed. Yet the difference between the Swedish and the American perspective becomes clear in the view of autism as a so-called 'superpower'. In Sweden, it is more common to feel that such labels can be experienced as intimidating and demoralising for someone with severe neuropsychiatric difficulties, someone who doesn't live up to the image of being a superhero. The autism spectrum is too wide for everyone to be able to relate to such an image. The simple answer is that autism can be both a blessing and a curse. The question is, what is more stigmatising — feeling like a victim of your own diagnosis or believing that autism can be turned into something positive?

§

When Tyla Grant from Britain started the YouTube channel *Autistic Tyla* at age 20 in 2018, she got thousands of subscribers. Today she is a staunch activist for autists' rights, posting videos about what she calls an autistic lifestyle. She talks about her life, promoting apps that can make the day-to-day easier, explaining the different aspects of autism, and combating prejudice.

Tyla and other autists on social media refer to their life strategy as 'unmasking'. Her goal is to quit masking and adapting entirely. She wants to live a true and authentic life. But changing one's behaviour is difficult and requires practice.

Another YouTuber, the American 27-year-old Jesslyn Craner, offers advice on how to unlearn and stop masking. With openness and ease, she shares concrete advice on how to realise whether one is masking even in front of oneself.

Embrace stimming and do it more at home, she says, extending her arms in a beautiful arc. Stim with me, she encourages her audience, streaming live on Instagram from her bedroom floor, surrounded by stim toys and swaying from side to side to the music.

I can't stop watching. I love her.

Craner's YouTube channel is aimed at autists who were diagnosed late in life, and her content is filled with hope and reassurance. In her videos, she acts like a sort of autistic influencer. There is no lack of darkness in what she shares about herself, but she is surrounded by an environment that seems like an autist's dream. She lives in a separate part of her parents' house that comes with a big garden, and in her room — which she has decorated in a style known as 'cottagecore' — she has created a rural, friendly world full of teacups, fairy lights, and house plants. A homemade patchwork quilt covers her bed, jewellery and flowery hair accessories hang from the shelves, and mounted on the wall is her grandmother's wedding photo. Here is her collection of Bowie vinyl and comic books; she has her library and a relaxation and stimming corner complete with fluffy cushions and a snack box.

On social media, Craner wants to create an inclusive community among autists and gather knowledge and tools for those, like herself, who weren't diagnosed as children. Since her diagnosis in adulthood, she has become whole and learnt to grow, she says. And I, who put too much faith in words, absorb every last one, thinking that while we wait for society and the neurotypicals to catch up, it's people like Jesslyn Craner — young, positive Americans with YouTube channels — who will keep us all afloat.

PEER PRESSURE

Name us the faithful.

ERIK AXEL KARLFELDT

In 2019, *Time* magazine named a young autistic woman its person of the year. With her enormous impact as a climate activist, Greta Thunberg has become a role model for autistic women and girls across the world, who finally have someone to identify with.

In an episode titled 'Anti-Greta', Swedish podcasters Alex Schulman and Sigge Eklund discuss Thunberg in relation to her polar opposite — the 19-year-old climate denier Naomi Seibt from Germany.

'I mean, she's like a part of the world,' Schulman says when he sees a picture of Seibt. 'She's blow-dried her hair, she's having coffee with friends. Greta lives apart from the world. How is she supposed to say something about the world when she's not a part of it?'

I puzzle over his choice of words. It's quick-witted and facetious, something he lets fly in the moment. But still. Why is he saying that Thunberg lives apart from the world? There is no doubt that he sympathises with her climate activism.

Even though Thunberg is the world's leading opinion-maker on the issue that will determine the fate of the world in our time, in Schulman's eyes she couldn't possibly understand the world, because she doesn't engage in normal teenage activities like blow-drying her hair and having coffee with friends. Choosing not to prioritise her appearance or social friendships is seen as so aberrant that such a young woman doesn't belong to this world.

Perhaps the choice of words strikes me because that is precisely how I feel sometimes — like I'm not connected to the rest of the world. No matter how hard I knock on the glass, I'm never let inside.

Thunberg herself has spoken about the bullying she was subjected to in school for being different. In the book *Our House Is on Fire*, her mother, Malena Ernman, describes the parents' shock as they visited their daughter at school and saw that none of the other children wanted to speak to her. Thunberg, however, was used to this treatment by her classmates.

People with autism make for good activists, says Thunberg. If it weren't for her condition, she wouldn't have noticed the climate crisis, wouldn't have grasped its gravity, and — most of all — wouldn't have taken action. Autists have no distance between what they say and what they do, she explains to *Teen Vogue*.

'Without my diagnosis, I also wouldn't have been such a nerd, and then I wouldn't have had the time and energy to look through the boring facts and still be interested.'

Of course, Greta would never care about a comparison with some 'Anti-Greta'. But the nature of her fame speaks to the difficulty that neurotypicals have understanding autists. Some want to paint her as calculating in her public persona. Many commentators can't grasp that she, unlike them, is driven by things other than attention.

I take refuge in Katarina A. Sörngård's *The Autism Handbook: strategies for an improved quality of life*. In it, I read about regular people: 'Many neurotypicals may struggle to understand that not everyone is like them.'

Sörngård writes that neurotypicals are scared of not fitting in in social settings and have been known to make great sacrifices so that they may be allowed into the group. They can be intolerant towards people who are different and stop at little to win the group's approval. 'They can claim to hold opinions they don't in order to be included, lie and withhold information, spend time with people they don't like, eat food they don't enjoy, dress in uncomfortable clothing.'

People with autism trust in themselves and exhibit great resilience against peer pressure. For them, it's often incomprehensible the way neurotypicals can be so preoccupied with others' opinions of them. They often have a strong sense of justice. Their stubbornness and ability to geek out mean they never give up. These are good qualities in an activist.

In the book *The Language of Poets, Children, and Fools*, I come across a chapter titled 'The Autistic Group'. At first, the thought amuses me. I picture a group of individuals, each one deeply absorbed in something — a book, a phone, or the activity of sorting. A silent, permissive collective where everyone is doing their own thing.

But that's not what the author Lisbet Palmgren means, I realise as I read on. To her, a collective autism describes a group so intensely tight-knit that it shuts other people out, almost like a sect or a filter bubble. The group is characterised by an exclusionary fanaticism and a shared self-image in which the only truth is its own norms. It's closed off to all other feelings, thoughts, and impressions than its own.

'Reality fades, neither pain nor self-criticism can reach us anymore; we are safe in our collective disengagement,' Palmgren writes.

I'm reminded of how rarely the adjective 'autistic' is used in a positive way.

But withdrawing is not the same as dissociating. That's an interpretation arising from the neurotypical experience of being ignored. Physical distance is not the same as spiritual distance. An autist can be present even if she doesn't make eye contact or have it in her to get together.

Being autistic means to enjoy being alone in an unchanging world. Most people seek the opposite: company and a sense of development. They feel stressed when nothing happens and gloomy from spending too much time alone.

The autist appears enigmatic and perhaps also threatening, because she doesn't shy away from other people's great terror: being set apart. She seeks what others fear. At least, that's what it looks like when she withdraws from the group. But she isn't actually distancing herself. She wants to be included, too; she just needs to gather her strength for a moment. Turning away, the autist looks, in the eyes of others, like someone who is rejecting her community.

The French philosopher Hélène Cixous writes that people hate exclusion because they are terrified of ending up there themselves, among the excluded.

'This is our emotional, our personal, and political problem, the fact that we can't bear exclusion. We are afraid of it, we hate to be separated,' says Cixous.

But shutting out the world isn't the same as rejecting others as less than. It simply means needing to be alone for a bit.

One can be separate from the collective yet a part of the world. For some people, standing on the sidelines is enough. Some of us are happier watching.

And group mentality can become destructive and turn into bullying, harassment, fanaticism, oppression, torture, and terror. Even a well-meaning cohesion rests on ideas about a common similarity. A person who withdraws is disruptive and sparks irritation in others.

Why is it so important to some people that everyone submit to the majority? Is it because of a need to control? To exercise power? Or is it a sign of fear? Jealousy?

Why can't neurotypical people be content with simply sitting and talking to each other? Why isn't it enough for them to be present together?

Instead, their relations have to be manifested in endless group activities on which the entire foundation for their affinity rests. If not everyone wants to take part in the snowball fight, go water skiing, or play Jenga, this amounts to a betrayal grave enough to threaten their very sense of belonging. The autist has ruined the mood.

In Sweden, there is a strong underlying conformism at the heart of our historic reforms for equality. While the intention has been good, ideas about equal rights have often been confused with notions about all people being the same — as though one presupposed the other.

When everyone is assumed to function the same way, anyone who is different becomes an anomaly and all but a provocation to the group. This triggers a need to cast the person who is different as a victim. Being allowed into the collective on the same terms isn't possible.

In her book *The Renaissance of the Immeasurable*, author and philosophy professor Jonna Bornemark describes how our time has lost itself in generalisations, rules, and abstractions and fallen out of touch with what it means to be human and alive. The pedants, in whose world we now live, have no ability to relate to unique, concrete situations and individuals, Bornemark argues. The more rigid systems we introduce, the less space there is for flexibility and understanding for those who fall outside the norm. And whose are the norms that permeate our rules and systems? Why, the neurotypicals', of course.

During the 2000s, the cult of measurability took hold in Swedish society. The pre-written manuals that now dominate the workplace assume that all employees are the same — and thus interchangeable. Their work is documented using forms that leave no space for anything beyond what has already been determined. That which used to be personal has been generalised in a societal development that doesn't benefit the autist.

In light of this development, it's easy to see why people who are different need their diagnoses. It's their only hope of being listened to. In a top-down system, that slip of paper turns into a tool for survival. With a diagnosis in black and white, adaptations might be made to meet your needs. Without it, you don't stand a chance.

Collectivism may take new expressions, but it continues to weed out those who don't conform.

In the first decades of the 20th century — during the very era when the Social Democratic Party laid the foundation for the Swedish welfare state — people who were perceived as deviants were stowed away at institutions. Sweden sterilised the highest number of people in Europe after Nazi Germany. Today, we look back in horror at the eugenics of the 20th century, when 63,000 people were sterilised in Sweden — mostly women. In around half of these cases, the surgery took place against the express will of the individual. Though it's questionable how free the choice was for those who consented.

Among those affected were people with mental illness or intellectual or physical disabilities — the so-called 'feeble-minded' or 'halfwits', and people with 'bodily defects' or 'disturbed souls' — as well as those in poor physical health, people with epilepsy, and transgender people. Society wanted to rid itself of individuals carrying 'bad genes'.

But people with a so-called 'asocial lifestyle' were sterilised, too. Who were they? Behaviour that was perceived to violate social norms and deviate from proper conduct was termed 'asocial'. Historical research has shown that it was enough to be seen as promiscuous or belong to the Roma 'traveller' community, also known as 'tinkers'. Anyone who didn't live up to society's idea of a proper life was considered biologically inferior. For people with epilepsy, a ban on marriage remained in place until 1969. They weren't allowed to marry and have children.

We live in a different time, yet people are still cast in the same mould. The management systems of our era create new demands for homogeneity.

It's not possible to understand people's unhappiness, exhaustion, and mental illness without analysing social developments and the reality they face in their everyday lives. There have always been autistic individuals, but the diagnosis only arises in the encounter with the world around them. The more streamlined society becomes, the more individuals who are different will stand out.

The fact that more people are diagnosed with autism today has to do with a growing awareness, but also with societal changes that have taken place in the recent past. One can point to a job market with tougher demands on employee versatility; a digital revolution in which the individual is expected to master more and more parts of life on their own; management by manual and automation where the requirements are locked in; ruthless rationalisation that eliminates slow-paced, predictable jobs; the return of daily or hourly wages with the rise of zero-hour contracts; changes to the educational system and pedagogy; and a heightened level of noise in public spaces.

There is something about Simone Weil. I read Katarina Frostenson's book *K*, in which she often returns to the French philosopher, mystic, and activist who died in 1943, a mere 34 years old. There is something familiar about the lines from Weil that Frostenson quotes. I can't put my finger on it. I note down two quotes in my phone and stare at them repeatedly.

'The person in a man is a thing in distress; it feels cold and is always looking for a warm shelter.'

And:

'To love a stranger as oneself implies the reverse: to love oneself as a stranger.'

The person *inside* the human being. It feels cold.

The quote about loving a stranger has been interpreted as expressing the insight that one can never fully know another human being. But it's the second half that draws me in, the part about loving oneself as a stranger. Why does Weil write that?

She wants to say something about accepting that which is strange within oneself. About the knowledge of — and reconciliation with — the stranger inside. And why is the other a stranger, too, instead of a neighbour? There is something like an urgent demand, perhaps also an accusation of guilt, in her reminder to the self to care more for the people around it.

My feeling was right. When I read about Weil's life, I immediately find information indicating that she was most likely autistic. The writer Rosemary Dinnage and the psychiatrist Michael Fitzgerald have, each in their own book, come to the same conclusion. The discovery is intoxicating; I feel like a detective. I knew it!

With the knowledge of Weil's likely autism in the back of my mind, her philosophical interest in the concept of attention becomes all but self-explanatory. The power of the soul lies in being attentive, she wrote. To her, this attention was key to both action and knowledge. She saw the highest degree of attention as a kind of prayer. Second only to guaranteeing freedom, she believed that the most important task of a government was to provide for an atmosphere of silence and attentiveness. A good society guards this silence and attentiveness so that its citizens can learn to express themselves.

Weil's books were published posthumously, and as a thinker she now enjoys a status that extends beyond the academic world, approaching that of Simone de Beauvoir. The most famous picture of her face — with her curly bob and round glasses — is reproduced in various artistic styles, like images of Che Guevara or Marilyn Monroe, and posted on Instagram captioned with selected quotes from her books.

Simone Weil lived her life in voluntary asceticism.

She was born in Paris in 1909, the second child in a Jewish family where the father was a doctor. She came into the world a month early and was a sickly and hypersensitive child. During her childhood, she was plagued by migraines and anorexia. She had motor difficulties involving her hands and struggled learning to write. Friends remember her sitting hunched over her papers with ink-stained hands, laboriously tracing the words, easily disturbed and always attentive to sounds and the goings-on around her.

Weil's mother said about her daughter that she was unspeakably stubborn, impossible to control.

In her early teens, she taught herself several languages, including classical Greek. She detested being touched and didn't even want to come into physical contact with her parents. At the age of ten, she began to demonstrate a strong sense of justice. She wouldn't stand for injustice and carefully followed the coverage of the Russian Revolution in the press. If a friend disappointed her, she ended the friendship abruptly.

In 1923, she enrolled at the Sorbonne as the sole woman in her class. She taught philosophy and art history at the girls' secondary school in Le Puy, and her students remembered a teacher who delivered her lectures in a monotonous voice without ever lifting her gaze from the text. She wrote newspaper articles about oppression and went on leave from the school to better understand the conditions of workers by taking a job on the assembly line in a car factory. She donated the pay she received to an unemployment fund.

When the Spanish Civil War broke out, she travelled to Spain to fight against the fascists. She learnt to use a gun, but struggled with her nearsightedness and failing motor skills. Soon, she was saved by her fearful parents, who came to pick her up. Around the same time, she began to open herself up to Christianity more and more. When World War II broke out, she escaped with her parents to southern France and lived in Marseille, where she wrote a great deal while waiting to go to the US. In her book *The Need for Roots*, she imagined the future of France.

Many of the stories about Weil are about her clumsiness. She is said to have dropped a suitcase with compromising documents about the French Resistance in the middle of the street and burnt herself badly by accidentally stepping into a vessel of boiling oil during the Spanish Civil War. She lived ascetically throughout her adult life, barely allowing herself anything to eat. At the age of 34, she was admitted to hospital with tuberculosis. On 24 August 1943, her heart could no longer hold out, and she died.

Weil's work was marked by her untiring pursuit of truth. She built her world of ideas on mentality and feeling, the spiritual communion between people. An important thought — her basic assumption — was that all people need a social context. Weil saw humanity's rootlessness as one of modernity's greatest troubles and emphasised belonging as a fundamental human need.

In *The Need for Roots*, she writes that 'a human being has roots by virtue of his real, active, and natural participation in the life of a community.'

These are the words of a person who knows what it means to feel alienated and who longs to be part of the community. Yet the autistic philosopher also puts great demands on this community. It has to be real and true, or else it is worthless.

In her books, Weil describes the autist's paradox: at the same time both longing for and shunning social life. It is often said about Weil that her experiences of the Spanish Civil War left her disappointed in the collective and the possibility of achieving justice within the framework of the political formations of her time. The insurrection in Spain, which ended in the fascist Francisco Franco rising to become its dictator, led her to relinquish all loyalty to any political party. But her aversion to the collective can also be read through the lens of the autist. Her scepticism runs deeper than her disappointment in the incompetence of political groups.

In her essay 'Human Personality', she writes: 'The collectivity is not only alien to the sacred, but it deludes us with a false imitation of it.'

The imitation of the feeling of sanctity that the collective provides is what is known as 'ersatz', Weil argues. Ersatz — the replacement of something true and real. She finds the part of the soul that says 'we' to be infinitely more dangerous than the part that says 'I'. Daring to go against the collective — 'the Great Beast' — was a virtue to Weil. Autists are bad politicians and impossible diplomats.

But if the false collective instils a false sense of security, what constitutes a true shared life according to Weil?

Her ideal is to reach the impersonal sphere. Here is where the sacred lives. And this, she says, is only possible through in solitude practising a rare kind of attention. It's not enough to practise external solitude — that is, to isolate. No, you must feel inner solitude, Weil demands. This means not experiencing oneself as part of a 'we' or a collective at all. The group can never be sacred, but neither can what Weil calls 'the personal'. The personal is that part of a human being which consists in errors, delusion, and sin. Weil appears to conceive of the personal as a mask, something transmutable that you can put on and take off — and therefore, not important.

That which is whole and true is impersonal, Weil argues. She wants to strip away people's veneers, move beyond the personal and the group. But what is this truth she finds there? To Weil, the sacred, the basis of human worth, the impersonal, is the human ability to suffer when experiencing bodily or spiritual harm. What remains is the trust of a child, the childlike core deep in every human heart that expects to be treated well, and thus protests when someone hurts it. That trust, that *expectation of goodness*, that part of the human heart which cries out in protest against evil, is eternal and unchanging in every human being. It is what we have in common.

Emily Dickinson described herself as a quiet earthquake. A 'Vesuvius at home', an inexorable volcano with hot lava coursing inside.

In descriptions of Dickinson's life and work, words like 'mysterious' and 'enigmatic' abound. She lived a secluded life in her father's house in New England and wrote her many poems, which weren't published until after her death in 1886. The last 15 years of her life, she rarely left home. When speaking to visitors, she would sometimes stand behind a closed door. With time, a romantic artist myth has been woven around her about an ethereal female figure who chose literature over reality.

What's 'enigmatic' about Dickinson appears to revolve around her self-inflicted isolation. Why didn't she ever marry? Why did she travel so little? In her poetry, she described the sea — but also wrote that she had never seen it.

In an extensive biography about Dickinson published in 1971, her life's trauma was described as never receiving enough love from her mother. Her mother's coldness supposedly triggered a nervous breakdown in the grown Emily, who withdrew from the world in order to dedicate herself solely to her poetry.

The problem with biographer John Cody's theory is that there are source materials in which Dickinson's contemporaries — friends and fellow poets — insist that she was 'born different', that her hypersensitivity, heightened presence, and odd behaviour had always been there. Cody remarks that this could only be true if Dickinson had some kind of 'new syndrome'. His comment was written in 1971, two decades before Asperger's syndrome was recognised as an official diagnosis.

Dickinson's life and poetry show clear signs of autism. She was hypersensitive to sensory input, covered her ears during thunder, suffered headaches from certain smells, didn't like to eat, and couldn't wear tight-fitting clothes. Yet her sensitive hearing also gave her a talent for music. She composed and played the piano, loved certain floral scents, and put a great deal of effort into her herbarium.

Socially, Dickinson struggled with boundaries. In her youth, she would suffocate her friends with intense declarations of love and demands for intimacy. In a letter to her sister-in-law from 1858, Dickinson fantasises about buying back the former's body after her death with her own blood, to keep in her garden or — preferably — in her bed. When she grew older, she withdrew from other people's company, but continued to write many letters. These were introverted and filled with philosophical musings, odd imagery, and twists of language.

In her book *Writers on the Spectrum*, the literature professor Julie Brown, who has researched the impact of autism on literary history, points out that Dickinson doesn't appear to be writing for a reader. Her poetry is fragmented and dissonant in a manner far ahead of her time. Reading her through an autistic lens, however, it's possible to imagine that she wrote more concretely than many have previously believed. Take, for example, the first stanza in poem 242:

> It is easy to work when the soul is at play —
> But when the soul is in pain —
> The hearing him put his playthings up
> Makes work difficult — then —

When the narrator's soul is at peace and she is happy, working is easy. But who is this 'him' that appears in the third line, with his 'playthings'?

Julie Brown makes the interpretation that the pronoun 'him' is Dickinson's soul, and ponders what the relation between play and work might have looked like for her. Others have read 'him' as a child who becomes a metaphor for the soul, with the implication that when the child inside suffers, the adult is unable to work. Personally, I read the last two lines of the poem as an expression of Dickinson's sensitivity to sound. Perhaps there was a boy with toys visiting the house, who disrupted her peace while writing.

Dickinson is one of the most read and loved poets in the US, and the analyses of her poetry are abundant. Her reinvention of the poetic form has been interpreted as a conscious political positioning, a way of exposing fundamental injustices through language. Feminist literary critics have argued that Dickinson intentionally deconstructed language, with the aim of stripping the patriarchy of its power.

The question is whether she really had such motives. Julie Brown doesn't think so; she believes Dickinson's unconventional style and stubborn independence was a consequence of her autism — though breaking with established form was indeed a conscious artistic choice. Dickinson's autism lent her enough eccentricity to be innovative and the courage to ignore other people's opinions. But she probably couldn't have written any other way.

In her poetry, Dickinson relied on metaphors and symbolism and explored themes close to autism. She knew that she was different and felt alienated from the rest of the world. Her sense of alienation expressed itself, for instance, through the repeated image of a boat or a swimmer bobbing up and down, alone on a vast sea. The latter is often present as an overwhelming, threatening force to struggle against and drown in, an enemy that the narrator can neither understand nor defeat. She uses universal imagery such as flowers, animals, and religious references, but also a personal kind that only she understood. Her poetry is often about death.

Emily Dickinson created a life together with her books and poems. In her poetry, she could express joy at the solitude she had chosen for herself — 'How happy is the little Stone / That rambles in the Road alone' — as well as a desire to become as 'independent as the Sun'.

I'm back in Falköping with Linn Sundberg, the artist with the trolls and the green paintings.

Ever since childhood, she has loved fairytales and built her own worlds, in her imagination or out of cardboard. As a child, she was often fearful and worried. She was close to tears and experienced strong separation anxiety, but could also lack boundaries. Sometimes she would walk up to strangers in town and give them a hug.

Linn didn't like playing in groups or being put in unexpected situations. Where her best friend lived, a couple of blocks away, there was a group of children who used to play together. Linn could never bike over there to see if anyone was outside and wanted to play; she always had to plan ahead and see preferably one but no more than two friends at a time. Everything needed to be predictable.

She got stressed and tense, and tried to direct the other children to create a sense of control.

'I've always felt most comfortable spending time with people who are younger or older than me. It's been hard to be with people my own age.'

Linn stayed home a lot and often played with her younger brother. She found it easier to be around boys. The social situations that arose were less difficult to navigate.

'I didn't have to think as much about accidentally saying something wrong or making someone upset. It was a recurring thing in lower secondary school. There'd be misunderstandings so often, it was like things went over my head all the time. I realised there were things going on in the air around me that I didn't grasp, but suddenly someone was upset. There were all these reactions I couldn't trace back to something I had said or done. There were lots of fights and trouble in my relationships with girls.'

As she grew older, social expectations intensified, the game became more complex, and Linn couldn't keep up at all.

In lower secondary school, Linn had a close friendship with a girl whose company she sought refuge in.

'I've always been the kind who likes to latch on to one person, who becomes like a safe place.'

But her friend struggled with poor mental health, and their friendship grew demanding. Often, the friend felt that Linn didn't live up to her expectations.

'Most of all in those conversations where you were supposed to talk about your feelings, and I sat there like a question mark, not knowing what to feel or talk about. Later, I've learnt that it was because I couldn't interpret emotions and bodily signals. I still struggle with it, but at that age I had no idea whatsoever. I didn't understand that I didn't understand what I felt. It was all confusion.'

The friend was often angry and disappointed. Linn didn't understand why and felt sad. They got into one fight after another. The relationship finally ended when their parents stepped in and told them they couldn't see each other anymore.

The friend made new friends, and people turned their backs on Linn when she walked past them in the school corridor. She was ostracised, which only increased her anxiety, and she suffered her first bout of depression.

In Linn's diagnosis, it says 'very high intelligence'. In school, she loved to read and picked up new languages with ease. But she couldn't concentrate on the subjects she thought were boring, like maths. Despite all the problems, she fought her way through school with good grades. She was fuelled by performance anxiety and got lucky with her teachers, who made concessions because they knew that she was struggling with mental illness.

When Linn was 14 years old, her mother brought home a book about girls with ADHD. But Linn wasn't receptive to the thought that she might have a neuropsychiatric condition, and another few years would go by before she realised.

Her depression and self-harming behaviour got in the way and obscured Linn's true problems. After the relationship with her best friend blew up, Linn started cutting herself.

'I had learnt that people did that to make it hurt less on the inside. And unfortunately, it worked really darn well.'

Linn isolated from her parents, siblings, and schoolmates, and spent her time online talking to others who were struggling, too.

'It probably wasn't very healthy, but at least it was some kind of community.'

No one close to her understood why she was feeling so intensely, panickingly unwell. The self-harm escalated. In school, she sought the company of boys and other ostracised girls. She tried to adapt in order to be accepted.

For a time, she started wearing make-up and tight-fitting clothes, which was enough for the girls in school to start calling her a slut. It didn't matter what she did, how she behaved or dressed — it was never right in the others' eyes. There was always something that wasn't good enough. Linn grew increasingly introverted. She started listening to angry and sad music that reflected the way she felt. She cut herself and dressed in black. She gave up and stopped trusting others. There were crisis meetings and anti-bullying teams at school, but the problems were too big and the help too late. The ball was already in motion.

In upper secondary school, she found a new group of friends, and life got better. But her depression and self-harm lingered, and other secondary symptoms emerged in the form of panic attacks, social anxiety, and an eating disorder.

She lost weight and ended up in the care of the child and adolescent psychiatric services. But no one realised that it was autism. Seen from the outside, she was still doing well in school. In addition to autism, Linn also has ADHD but has never been particularly hyperactive. And conditioned to look for the more extroverted behaviour typically seen in boys, the psychiatric services failed to make that diagnosis, too. Instead, they concluded that she suffered from depression and panic attacks. The doctor wanted to prescribe antidepressants, but Linn refused. She didn't want any pills. They let her come in for a few appointments with a therapist, but these led nowhere.

'It's a problem when you're only focused on treating the symptoms — you can keep doing that forever.'

Linn has always been good at imitating, taking on a personality adapted to the people she is with, both in friendships and in love.

In upper secondary school, she buckled under the weight of her own performance demands; all the while, her sensitivity to sensory input added to the distress of being at school. She skipped class a lot and struggled to keep her head above water. On her lunch break, she would often go to a friend's house to sleep on the couch for an hour.

'I fell asleep in school all the time. For a while there, it turned into a game — I'd study the impressions on my forehead to figure out where I'd fallen asleep. "Okay, now there are squares, that's the keyboard in the computer room."'

After managing to graduate with decent grades, she was exhausted. She wasn't ready for adult life, and her anxiety prevented her from applying for jobs. Yet she managed to land a temporary position as a youth leader with the Equmenia Christian youth ministry. Linn had grown up within the Mission Covenant Church of Sweden, where her mother had been a choir director, so the church was a safe space for her. She worked with Equmenia for just under a year. The demands were low and the days short. During this period, her anxiety eased. But she could still feel that something was wrong inside — even though she was doing better, she couldn't make life work. A teacher on a course she took scolded her for doodling during a lecture. The teacher thought she wasn't listening, but Linn tried to explain that she couldn't follow along with what was being said if she wasn't allowed to do something with her hands in the meantime.

'There was a moment when the teacher said: "Focus, Linn, stay with us!" I got angry and repeated the last three sentences he had spoken word for word.'

She moved to another town and started applying for jobs there, but felt anxious and weak. Her confidence sank as she missed one interview after another. She started googling ADHD, went to her doctor, and finally got referred for an assessment.

Through the Public Employment Service, she participated in a work-training scheme at a charity shop, and liked it, but the exhaustion still came. Her eating and sleeping habits began to suffer. Her occupational therapist at the Public Employment Service knew that Linn was waiting to do her psychological assessment but still felt that she had an attitude problem and wasn't trying hard enough.

'That's frustrating to be told when you are constantly struggling and labouring to make life work — just to do laundry and have something clean to wear, make sure to eat something other than sandwiches, drink water, and clean so that you're not living in unsanitary conditions. My occupational therapist was a little older, so it was completely hopeless. She was very strict and wanted me to work full-time, but I crashed at 75 per cent and had to drop everything, otherwise I would've had to be committed. You just really want to be able to do it. You really want to live up to those expectations.'

After a two-year-long wait, the assessment finally happened. When Linn was 22 years old, in the spring of 2012, she was diagnosed with autism level 1 and ADHD.

'It was such a relief. It was an answer and confirmation that my brain works differently and that it's not me who is bad. I've always thought that I just suck at being human. That I just happen to be a particularly crappy one.'

Linn has lived a destructive life, self-harming and self-medicating, which escalated when her mother suddenly passed away. She moved cities, left a bad relationship, and managed to free herself of her addiction.

The way her strengths have tended to obscure her difficulties has been a constant frustration.

'If I hadn't been so smart, they might have noticed something sooner. Intelligence can compensate for so much. When others perceive you as intellectually clever, they struggle to understand that you can have all these problems. It doesn't add up that someone who is good at thinking can fail so utterly at things that are easy for others.'

Thanks to the art gallery, Linn has found new meaning in life and sees a brighter future ahead. She wants to be part of growing the gallery's artistic activities and to continue with her own art while also teaching others — give lectures, perhaps; organise workshops.

'I want to work with art and information dissemination, using the creativity and energy in my special interests to create my own job. My dream is to be able to create the contexts I want to be in. One important aspect is getting to share it with other people. I have no interest in just making my own art.'

She dreams of putting on an exhibition at the gallery with artworks by autistic artists.

'I hope I'll continue to develop towards feeling better, so that I can do more and contribute to other people's lives and to society. But it's taken a long time to get to a point where I can have a positive outlook on the future.'

I LOCK MY DOOR
UPON MYSELF

It took a long time before I saw my husband, that he
existed in the physical world.

AUTISTIC WOMAN, INTERVIEWED IN

AUTISM: RELATIONSHIPS AND SEXUALITY BY GUNILLA GERLAND

How do you create a lasting romantic relationship when you have a
big need for alone time, are not the caring type, can't lie, and struggle
to pick up on signals from your partner? For female autists, love is
perhaps even trickier, since expectations on women are high: they are
considered more emotionally intelligent, intuitive, and empathetic, and
in heterosexual relationships are often principally responsible for the
couple's social life.

In the Facebook group Neurotypical Partners of Autistic People,
neurotypical individuals — mostly Americans — have created a safe
space where they can exchange experiences of living with an autist. The
group consists almost exclusively of women forced to act as mothers and

maids to their tactless autistic men who don't lift a useful finger around the home. Partners complaining about their autistic women are rare in the group; they barely exist.

But in the Netflix series *Love on the Spectrum*, autistic women are represented. It's a modern and warm-hearted Australian reality show that follows the awkward attempts of a few young adults trying to find love. All the participants on the show are autists and only date other autists.

'What's it like for you being a girl on the spectrum?' the producer asks a participant named Olivia.

'Extremely difficult, considering that there's no girl criteria,' she replies. 'It's only boy. So you get assessed on how male you are.'

On the show, most attempts at romance end in friendship. The participants both want and don't want to get closer. Special interests collide. A girl brings her Nintendo Switch to a dinner date so she will have something to do at the restaurant. A guy bores his date with an endless monologue about dinosaurs. Their parents try hard to teach them to be polite, reminding them to listen to the other person and ask follow-up questions to keep the conversation going.

But some of the couples do work out, and take solace in understanding each other. When the 21-year-old Jimmy breaks down over his socks being the wrong colour ahead of a dinner, his partner Sharnae calmly hands him a Rubik's cube to settle his nerves. Then she goes out with him to buy new socks.

In 2012, the British autism researcher Damian Milton — who is an autist, too — introduced an idea that he called the 'double empathy problem'. His assumption was that autistic people don't actually suffer from social difficulties, they simply communicate better with others who think like them. The same is true of neurotypicals.

During an experiment at the University of Edinburgh in 2019 conducted by Catherine Crompton, participants were divided into

three groups and instructed to play a round of telephone. One group
consisted solely of autists, another solely of non-autists, and the third
was mixed.

In two of the groups, the game worked well. In both the autistic
and the non-autistic groups, the whispered message travelled along
the chain of participants almost unchanged from start to finish. In the
mixed group, it worked less well. Huge misunderstandings arose during
the course of the whispering, and by the time the game was over the
original sentence had become another one entirely.

The results indicate that both autists and non-autists work best with
others of the same kind. When they come together, communication
fails. It's a somewhat bleak conclusion, since the consequence would be
some kind of separatism.

> I lock my door upon myself,
> And bar them out; but who shall wall
> Self from myself, most loathed of all?
> [...] God harden me against myself,
> This coward with pathetic voice
> Who craves for ease, and rest, and joys

From 'Who Shall Deliver Me?' (1866) by Christina Rossetti

The painting *I Lock My Door upon Myself* from 1891 by the Belgian
artist Fernand Khnopff hangs in a museum in Munich. The title has
been borrowed from Christina Rossetti's poem 'Who Shall Deliver
Me?', a biblically inspired text about an inner struggle from which God
is the only salvation.

The painting shows a redheaded woman sitting by a table, resting
her chin on her hands. Her gaze is bright and turned inwards. She
looks past the observer, but the expression on her face is calm and

shows no signs of angst. She appears at peace in her contemplation. On a shelf next to the woman is a bust of the Greek god of sleep, Hypnos. In the foreground are three red, wilting lilies. To the right of the woman is a painting within the painting: a lone, dark figure in an urban environment.

Christina Rossetti was the sister of the Pre-Raphaelite artist Dante Gabriel Rossetti, whom Fernand Khnopff admired. But Khnopff himself belonged to the Symbolists, who painted humanity's inner world. They wanted to portray ideas and moods. The feelings manifested on the canvas were supposed to say something about a grander state. The Symbolists were interested in ambiguity — in poetry, fantasy, and dreams.

As a reaction to the rapid industrialisation and urbanisation of its time, late 19th-century art looked inwards, at the human psyche.

The painting has been interpreted as portraying a turning away from the world, something Khnopff did himself, building a fort-like home in Brussels intended as a bastion against what he perceived to be a vulgar outside world.

But who was the enigmatic woman? Barely a century after it was painted, the New York–based publisher Ecco Press began publishing a series of texts inspired by visual artworks. The author Joyce Carol Oates chose Khnopff's painting.

In Oates's novella *I Lock My Door upon Myself* from 1990, the name of the redheaded main character is Calla Honeystone. The year is 1912 in Chautauqua County, Upstate New York, and Calla — who is named after a funeral flower — needs no one's company. As a child, she speaks of herself in the third person. She prefers wandering the woods alone rather than going to school or spending time with her family. She is fully self-sufficient. In adulthood, she turns away from her husband, parents, and children.

Behind Calla's back, people are talking. In the neighbourhood, they are saying that she has been 'touched in the head'. Calla hears the gossip and it makes her both furious and strangely content. She imagines that it's God who has touched her head, and that it means she is destined for great things.

On one of her walks, Calla meets a man with whom she falls violently in love. She cheats on her husband, but is punished by losing her love. The man drowns in a waterfall.

After his death, Calla stays inside for 55 years.

Her mantra is: 'I do what I do, what I do is what I wanted to have done' and 'My self is all to me. I don't have any need of you.'

Oates's novella has been read as a story about self-deception, with Calla's motive as its inherent mystery. Why does such a powerful person voluntarily isolate herself? Has her heart been broken — has she been crushed by her lost love? Or is the isolation like time spent in a convent, where she is choosing God over her own desires?

Oates offers no clear answer as to why Calla locks her door upon herself. But it's only a mystery to those who consider voluntary solitude as strange and abnormal.

It's the 1980s and I'm sitting in a red velvet chair at the opera with my parents. I'm hot. My plaid skirt in lined flannel is too wide around the waist and gets twisted every time I move. Its folds chafe, and the flannel creates an unnerving friction against the bristly velvet of the chair.

We are waiting for the ballet *Coppélia* to begin. I'm hoping I will get a chocolate pastry in the intermission. At the cinema, Dad and I usually bet on whether the curtain will be raised or pulled to the side. But here at the opera, I have been before — so when it rises quickly and soundlessly, I'm prepared.

The stage is a village square where the dollmaker and inventor Dr Coppelius lives. On the balcony of his house sits a young, rosy-cheeked woman reading a book. A male dancer who seems to be the hero of the story tries in vain to get her attention. Franz, as he is called, performs a pas seul and is soon joined by more male dancers gazing up at the balcony with big eyes. But the young woman sits motionless with her book, staring straight ahead. She doesn't see them.

The girl is a mechanical doll: Coppélia. Dad explains that Franz becomes so taken with the doll that he forsakes his human fiancée Swanhilda. Told in parallel is the story about the dollmaker Coppelius's obsession with his creation, and his dream of turning the doll into a living creature. But Coppélia cannot be brought to life; she is and remains a doll. And in the end, Franz chooses the real-life Swanhilda. He makes the wrong choice, I think from my seat in the audience. The doll is my favourite.

The comic ballet *Coppélia*, set to music by Léo Delibes, first premiered in Paris in 1870. The victory of the human over the soulless doll is made complete in the final scene when the two lovers are reunited in a pas de deux all the while a lifeless Coppélia is carried off the stage.

The libretto about the unfeeling doll and the insidious dollmaker is based on the short story 'The Sandman' by E.T.A. Hoffmann. Hoffmann was a science-fiction pioneer who liked to write fairytales for adults about the line between human and machine, where the main character lived in the borderland between fantasy and reality.

When Sigmund Freud wrote his famous essay on the concept of *das Unheimliche*, he based it in part on his own reading of 'The Sandman'.

In the short story, the character Nathanael falls in love with a doll, Olimpia. The story also contains a terrifying creature threatening to claw out the eyes of little children. Freud argues that 'The Sandman' arouses *unheimliche* feelings in the reader and analyses the fear of losing one's eyes as an expression of Nathanael's castration anxiety.

A common feminist critique aimed at Freud's reading of 'The Sandman' is that he overlooks the doll Olimpia. This, researcher Jutta Emma Fortin believes, is because the doll doesn't awaken any particular feelings of discomfort in Freud, who sees her through Nathanael's male gaze. And to him, she is as real as any woman.

Fortin sees Nathanael's fixation with the doll and his inability to have a relationship with a real, independent woman as an expression of men's desire to control women.

In the story, the quiet, will-less doll Olimpia is an extension of Nathanael himself, an empty vessel for him to fill with his needs and desires.

Towards the end of the 16th century in Padua, Italy, the anatomy professor Hieronymus Fabricius built a jointed anatomical doll. Fabricius re-imagined the human body as a set of metal pieces, rivets, and screws.

In 18th-century France, the engineer and inventor Jacques de Vaucanson constructed so-called 'biomechanical automatons': one that could play the tambourine, a flautist that breathed of its own accord, and a duck with 800 movable parts that could flap its wings, lift its legs, feed, quack, and shake its tail feathers. The audience was entranced.

In the mid-1800s, a doll went on sale in the US and became a sensation. Autoperipatetikos could walk with the help of an ingenious clockwork mechanism hidden underneath her skirt.

In his stories, E.T.A. Hoffmann captures this fascination with the boundary between creature and object, man and machine. People's admiration for fantastical automatons carrying out tasks almost as though they were alive was enormous. They liked to be entertained by mechanical figures performing for them.

In the 1950s, French director Robert Bresson began making films populated with human 'automatons'. Instead of 'actors', he called them 'models'. His method was to have them repeat each line and movement so many times that it wore them out, which made their actions automatic. The actors would eventually forget their lines and movements so that these happened unthinkingly. Only then, Bresson imagined, did the scene become true — as in real life. As a director, he wanted to eliminate all expressions of emotion in the actors; his goal was 'being' instead of 'seeming'.

In a book about his method, he writes: 'Models who have become automatic (everything weighed, measured, timed, repeated ten, twenty times) and are then dropped in the medium of the events of your film — their relations with the objects and persons around them will be *right*, because they will not be *thought*.'

Bresson saw repetition as a fundamental part of life. He imagined that almost everything people do and feel is governed by habit and automatism: 'Nine-tenths of our movements obey habit and automatism. It is anti-nature to subordinate them to will and to thought.'

Here, Bresson couched his artistic dreams of authenticity in scientific assumptions about human nature. He expressed a belief that a human being who thinks her way through life and the day-to-day is going against nature. But those of us who do are no less authentic, we simply function differently.

During the ballet performance of *Coppélia* at the opera, something happened in me. The doll became the main character. In me, she kindled no uncanny feelings of discomfort. On the contrary, she felt instantly familiar. I identified with her. She sat reading on the balcony and did as she pleased.

As a child, I didn't grasp that the doll might be an oppressed victim in the hands of a man, of course. My experience mostly had to do with the kind of miracle that only the performing arts can produce: the doll came to life in my eyes because she was being played by a living person. There and then, in that space, I saw with my own eyes that she was alive as she danced across the stage with jerky movements. She couldn't be reduced to an empty reflection, or a surface for other people's projections; I could see that she was a person. I witnessed it.

The doll that comes between a pair of human lovers is only one in a string of supernatural female creatures in romantic 19th-century ballet, and *Coppélia* wasn't my only love affair on the stage. I also saw nymphs, fairies, shadows, elves, swans, and sylphs, and was captivated by these odd creatures' alienation. The stories told in classical ballet were populated by strange, mysterious, offbeat women portrayed in their own right in a way that was rare in the children's culture of the 1980s, where the ideal was an adventurous tomboy.

The ballerinas seemed to float weightlessly, but even the child in the flannel skirt could see that their lightness of foot required enormous effort. From my seat in the audience, I saw their thigh muscles working, I saw that the ballerinas commanded an immense force and that they were always the main characters of their story. The male dancers mostly moved behind them, occasionally offering a supporting arm.

The ballerinas in the ballets of the 19th century sought revenge by dancing deceitful men to their deaths. They ignored, tricked, and pined or died for their suitors. They were the underworldly spirits of young women who had been betrayed before their wedding, like in *Giselle* (in Mats Ek's version from 1982, the spirits are female inmates at a mental hospital instead); or spirits of the forest, like the elusive sylph in *La Sylphide*. They challenged the order of things and were deeply unreliable.

The doll, though controlled by the dollmaker, seemed to have an inviolable inside and her own free will. She didn't care about the men around her. The creatures of the underworld lived their own lives in the shadows but came out and bothered people as they pleased.

I was drawn to the darkness of these stories, concealed under what seemed light and sheer on the surface.

What's more, the ballet offered a space free from spoken language.

The language of dance showed that it was possible to communicate beyond words. The movements of the dancers, their postures, gestures, and mimes, gave me a sense of clarity. This, I understood. The discipline, control, and willpower of the intense training — that which I would later realise gave classical ballet its bad reputation — also appealed to me. In my eyes, the strict rules offered safety; there was a clear right and wrong way to dance. I started taking lessons, but couldn't get out of my own head and didn't find the courage to try my body's limits. I preferred to be a spectator.

I still go to the ballet. In a version of *Coppélia* from 2019, the doll has been exchanged for an android with artificial intelligence.

INSULA

One of the jurors had a pencil that squeaked. This of course, Alice could not stand, and she went round the court and got behind him, and very soon found an opportunity of taking it away.

LEWIS CARROLL, *ALICE'S ADVENTURES IN WONDERLAND*

The Irish psychiatrist Michael Fitzgerald has researched the lives of famous historical individuals and, with the help of source materials such as biographies, diaries, letters, testimonials from relatives, and contemporaneous medical assessments, has tried to determine whether there are signs that the person might have received an autism diagnosis had they been alive today. His book *The Genesis of Artistic Creativity: Asperger's syndrome and the arts* features 20 men and one woman — the philosopher Simone Weil.

Found here is also the male author who wrote literary history's most famous depiction of a young girl lost in a strange, mystifying world. After improvising the tale on a rowing trip, Lewis Carroll wrote down *Alice's Adventures in Wonderland* for his good friend's daughter Alice Liddell. The book, which is filled with humour, riddles, and nonsense, marked his debut as an author. It's packed with hidden quotes, allusions, proverbs, parody and satire of other people's work, nursery rhymes, poems, and fairytales. Without a critical apparatus of footnotes, the many layers of reference are hard to penetrate for today's readers. Carroll constructed quirky, intricate puns and used a type of collage technique, where all the many books he had read spilled out onto the pages.

Lewis Carroll, whose real name was Charles Lutwidge Dodgson, wanted to be invisible to the world. He hid behind his pseudonym and lived a secluded life in Oxford. His first 11 years of life he spent almost completely isolated in his parents' rectory in the English countryside. Young Charles could often be found stretched out on the grass in the garden, writing. He counted snails and toads among his friends. At boarding school, he was bullied, but life became easier once he went on to university. After studying mathematics at Oxford, he stayed on as a tutor. A structured, quiet life focused on intellectual labour suited him.

Those who met him saw a black-clad man strictly bound by his routines who rarely laughed, was extremely sensitive to draughts, and brewed his own tea according to a set ritual during which he swung the teapot back and forth for exactly ten minutes in order to achieve the perfect flavour. He was described as a quiet and uncompromising bachelor, only capable of speaking about topics that interested him — including logic, time, mathematics, and puzzles. As a lecturer, he was hopeless and didn't get through to his students. Yet he showed great discipline in his work, disliked interruptions, and often forgot to eat.

There are psychoanalytic readings of *Alice's Adventures in Wonderland* that argue that the book reflects Carroll's fear of sex. Yet I think — as does literary scholar Julie Brown — that he writes this way, about these things, because of his autism.

In a single text, Carroll leapt from the Victorian era into postmodernism, writes Brown in her book *Writers on the Spectrum*, and that text was *Alice's Adventures in Wonderland*.

It's a story without traditional dramaturgy. In Wonderland, things happen haphazardly. There is no cause and effect; events are not organised in a forward movement where one thing leads to another. If one were to throw the chapters of the book into the air and let them land in a completely different order, it wouldn't change the story much.

It's not the main character, Alice, who propels the story onwards. She has no way of influencing those she meets in Wonderland, nor do they influence her. There is no frame narrative to speak of. There is no change in Alice, and the story has no resolution; it simply ends. When she finally wakes, it has all been a dream.

Alice never finds out what the White Rabbit is late for; she encounters two mice telling stories, the ends of which she never gets to hear; and the puppy that appears and plays with her never comes back.

Wonderland is a world of singularities, where Alice wanders between events and adventures on a journey without any abstract driving force such as love, faith, or loyalty. There is no bigger story, no framework to hold the events of the book together — they just happen.

The shifts in time and space strike her suddenly and mercilessly, and Alice is alternately frightened, disoriented, and curious. She doesn't have time to reflect on what is happening to her before she is thrown into something new. The moment is all there is. In the sequel, *Through the Looking-Glass, and What Alice Found There*, even time itself begins to move backwards.

Alice gets lost and loses touch with parts of her body as it alternately shrinks and grows. She tries hard to understand the strange characters she meets but fails — wishing the animals weren't so easily insulted — and constantly feels lonely.

She accidentally offends birds and mice by talking about her cat, not realising that she is scaring them. She always speaks the truth when questioned and is constantly tested by everyone she meets. They want her to solve riddles, answer questions, read verses, and tell stories, all at a rapid, cranked-up pace. She is surrounded by a grinning madness.

Alice attends a tea party, a game of croquet, and a trial — but never understands the codes or the rules of the game in any of the settings. Everything is confusing, both to her and to the characters she meets. Wordplay follows on literal interpretations, homonyms, and semantic misunderstandings.

In *Through the Looking-Glass*, the Caterpillar, the Cheshire Cat, and Humpty Dumpty all show their own signs of autism. The Caterpillar is a diligent fault-finder, continually objecting; Humpty Dumpty is face blind and, much like the Frog Footman, avoids eye contact; both Humpty Dumpty and the Cheshire Cat interpret language literally. The mouse from the pool of tears tries to dry the wet animals with the driest story it knows, about William the Conqueror.

Lewis Carroll's books about Alice are some of the most well-quoted and reinterpreted works in literary history, inspiring many artists, filmmakers, and authors. In her autobiographical poetry collection *The Autistic Alice*, the British poet Joanne Limburg, who grew up with undiagnosed autism, has homed in on Alice's autistic traits and turned her into an alter ego. In scenes from the Wonderland of Limburg's own childhood, the narrator tries to crack the impossible code of reality but is always getting it wrong. She is adrift in a haphazard reality, and the admonitions of the adult voices echo through the poems. She is the big Alice who feels hopelessly awkward yet also a little superior; she shrinks and turns into the small Alice who wants to disappear.

The poems reveal a human being striving for truth and depth, who thinks you shouldn't be allowed to call something an answer unless it is complete.

When my husband and I have been married for four years, we decide to return to the Italian island where we had our wedding and which I visited as a child. We have had a baby, and in the space where his parental leave overlaps with mine, we take our trip. I stand on the deck of the ferry, gripping the cold, oily railing. In front of me, the island rises out of the sea. Its hillsides are wrapped in a blanket of coniferous trees, and the waves break against rocks coloured rusty by the metals in the earth.

It's the same ferry as in the 1980s, a small passenger ship called *Planasia*. More than 30 years have passed since I first came here, but the ship is the same. How long does a ferry last?

Plump, warm raindrops hit the harbour square as I run to the bakery with the baby pressed against my chest to buy an almond cake for my husband's birthday. I don't know if he wants it. He has changed. Something is different ever since his mother died.

We spend more than a month on the island, driving all over. It belongs to us. We conquer every village. Every promontory, church, and bar is ours.

The restaurants are barred up and the tourists have gone home, the sailboats have left the harbour. It's the off-season, and time has slowed down. We have dinner at the roadside eatery — strange, boiled meat dishes with lemon halves and endive leaves — laughing at the Mussolini labels on the wine bottles on the shelves.

We bring our baby on a walk up to a limestone church in the mountains, taking turns to carry him when the road gets too stony and narrow, forcing us to leave the pram. The church is closed. We try to peer inside through the cracks in the wooden door, but it's pitch-black in there. Outside is a small terrace. On each side, closing in on us, are the mountains. We look out over the valley. A mouflon sheep bleats in the distance. Somewhere far away in the woods, there is a rustling. A nightingale sings. Our son is five months old, asleep against his dad's shoulder.

We are standing atop a mountain rising from the bottom of the sea. Speaking to each other is impossible. It's as though we are cursed. And yet life is easier here than when we return home to Stockholm, no longer under the island's protection. He isn't happy on parental leave, and I'm still stricken from giving birth. He wants to move again and again. But moving makes me so uneasy that I don't get involved at all, leaving him to do everything because I don't actually want to move even though I don't realise it. I can't make myself understood.

He is never on time, and I can't stand it. My anxiety claws at me, and I make a big fuss every time. He grows more and more silent but continues to be late. Things disappear from our home, forgotten or lost, and I can't stand this either. It doesn't bother him. 'I'll buy a new one,' he says simply, while I'm in a state of dissolution. I want to know where things are. He sighs at my piles of books and paper but doesn't understand that I know in my head exactly where everything is. Nothing must be shifted around. He changes plans and agreements, and it makes me begin to doubt whether his word means anything to him.

Our fights are incomprehensible to me — I love him so much. He is like a stone statue that I rush into headfirst, over and over again. When I speak, he doesn't understand that I mean every word I say. He thinks that I mean something else, that there is a hidden meaning behind my words, or that I'm exaggerating. But for the most part, he says very little. About his own feelings, he says nothing at all. He simply presses onwards through the day-to-day. He tries harder than I do.

I wrap myself in barbed wire. I become reluctant to all his suggestions. Because I don't feel when I'm hungry or thirsty, every interruption for a meal becomes an annoyance. I don't want to be interrupted and forced to think about something else. I'm fully absorbed in taking care of our child; taking in myself, too, becomes overwhelming. I rage at his back when he spends long stretches of time cooking by the stove, even though he is doing it for us. When our life together can no longer consist in play, we can't make it work.

Differences that we used to be able to counter become unmanageable. 'That's what everyone else does,' he says to me sometimes. It drives me crazy.

'I don't care what everyone else does!' I shout back.

SCHOOL AND WORK

I'm not sick, not sick
No, I'm not sick, not sick
I'm just tired, so infinitely tired
But I'm not sick, not sick

BJÖRN AFZELIUS, 'THE BALLAD ABOUT K'

Carolina Alexandrou in Rågsved, who loves Marilyn Monroe, has struggled to find her place professionally. In upper secondary school, she started working at a burger chain. One day, her manager asked her to go into the storeroom to get something. Carolina didn't understand what he meant.

'It was so messy in that room. I didn't dare ask — he had a very brusque way about him.'

Carolina tried to guess what her boss wanted. She grabbed a thing at random from the storeroom and handed it over. He was livid.

'"Are you completely retarded?" he asked me. I got really sad.'

Shortly after, she quit working at the burger place.

A few years later, she took a job at a preschool. The hustle and bustle around all the little children overwhelmed her. She had no energy.

One time, she sank down onto a couch to get a moment's rest. Her co-workers went to their boss and said that she had fallen asleep on the job. It wasn't true, but the manager believed them, and Carolina's zero-hour contract wasn't extended.

She trained as a nursing assistant and got a job at a care home for people with dementia in Huddinge, just outside of Stockholm. One day, the manager called her into her office and told Carolina that her colleagues said she couldn't work with others and wasn't doing her job. Carolina was shocked.

'To me they had said I was doing great. There was no truth in what they said. I felt like I was running around all the time — there is no end of things to do at a care home for people with dementia. But my boss chose to believe them.'

Carolina found out that her probationary employment was being terminated. Her boss didn't want to hear her version, trusting instead in her colleagues' accusations. She got no explanation as to how she had supposedly failed to do her job, despite asking for one. That is when she got angry.

'I told my boss straight up: "You're so fucking fake." And I stand by that. I couldn't keep it in. She wanted to fire me on the spot, but I stood my ground and said that I would finish my hours first, which I did. Then I went home.'

If someone treats her badly, she speaks up. When that happens, it doesn't matter who she is talking to.

Later, when Carolina applied for another job within the psychiatric services, she was given a poor reference by a previous employer and didn't get the job. Afterwards, she fell into depression and ended up on disability support.

For more than ten years, Carolina has had a steady stream of temporary employment contracts within child and elderly care as well as hospitality. Over and over again, she has been told by her superiors that it's not working, without understanding why. Sometimes she has left a job after feeling ill-treated or overwhelmed by stress.

'I've not been able to hold down a job. There has always been discord in the workplace. The boss has sat me down to tell me that I can't work together with others and that my colleagues have been saying things about me. And when that happens, I've wondered why they can't just come up and say it to my face. Like, stand up and tell it like it is. I would've had more respect for that. It felt like they were going behind my back, trying to push me out.'

Eventually, her anxiety and depression got so severe that she turned to psychiatry for help. At the age of 30, she was diagnosed with autism. Finally, it was as like something fell into place. After her diagnosis, life got better. Only then did she understand herself and realise that the jobs she'd had were unsuitable for a person who is hypersensitive to sensory stimuli. Stressful industries with high noise levels and many short social interactions are a bad fit for an autist.

'It feels like my true self has come out. I'm more alive now.'

But she has also been met with scepticism — people telling her that she doesn't seem autistic. They mean well, but don't understand that Carolina isn't ashamed of her diagnosis.

'When people say that, I begin to doubt myself and think: "No, maybe I don't have autism. Maybe I'm just lazy and stupid." But I know how hard I've fought. And that's not a lazy person.'

Today, Carolina is doing work training at a publishing company. Sitting in front of a computer fits her perfectly. She loves to write, but doesn't know how long she will be allowed to stay. Sometimes she despairs at the thought of finding her path professionally. When she reads job ads, she feels dispirited.

'"As a person, you are extroverted, super social, flexible, stress resistant, able to keep many balls in the air," blah, blah, blah. Seriously? Who has all these qualities they're looking for? Why should everyone be the same? Why not look for someone who is introverted, shy, thorough, structured, and focused on doing their job instead of gabbing away all the time? Why does everyone always have to be so bloody social?'

Carolina wants to work and make money, not be on disability support. But most officers at the Public Employment Service lack knowledge about autism, she says. They want you to apply for all kinds of jobs. Many of the industries where it's easiest to get a job are also the worst suited for autists.

'But we have a lot to contribute on the job market if we're given the right opportunities. We see things that neurotypicals don't. But many employers don't understand that. One of my case officers at the Public Employment Service called my diagnosis a disease. They need to be educated. And they should individualise more and realise that people are different.'

On the Swedish public-broadcasting TV show *Your Brain*, hosted by the author and psychiatrist Anders Hansen, there is a segment with an autistic woman who has found her ideal workplace. Jessica Dagerhamn, who has a PhD in infection biology, is very skilled at quickly reading summaries of scientific literature — so-called 'abstracts' — and identifying the most important content.

Dagerhamn believes this strength is tied to her autism. When she looks at a text, she can swiftly determine what parts are relevant. Certain words sort of pop out from the page and are more clearly visible, she explains.

In the TV segment, Dagerhamn is filmed in front of her computer at her workplace. The footage is riddled with visual stereotypes about autists. The camera lingers on a close-up of Dagerhamn's eyes, at the same time as animated letters quickly flash across the screen. Playing in the background is Hans Zimmer's dramatic soundtrack to the science-fiction film *Interstellar*. She reads so fast, it's inhuman.

Dagerhamn has been lucky enough to be matched with a broad-minded supervisor who knows to take advantage of her special skills by letting her focus on her expertise. In the workplace, she is allowed to sit in a quiet section for people who need more seclusion. Her boss says that she is one of his best hires; no one is more efficient. While he can read 200 abstracts in a day, she can do 1,000 in four hours.

Dagerhamn says that she thinks she has had it easier than others with neuropsychiatric diagnoses because she has a doctorate. When she mentions her diagnosis, she doesn't have to worry that people will think she is less intelligent.

'What do you feel is the biggest struggle, today?' Anders Hansen asks.

'All the other stuff,' Dagerhamn replies. 'I have kids. There's cooking, laundry, grocery shopping, and cleaning to do. Reading scientific texts, understanding — that's easy. Running a home isn't easy — it's barely doable.'

Ida Hallin Mellwing in Valdemarsvik, the mother with young children and the schedule of chores, works as a cleaner a few hours a week. The job suits her. She gets to meet people at the same time as she can work alone and have her own routines. She is thorough, and notices little details that other people miss.

'I'm a proud cleaner. I like my job, and I know that I'm good at it.'

After secondary school, Ida got a few different internships with the help of the Public Employment Service, including in a flower shop and a second-hand shop. She was good at keeping things in order and making it look nice on the shelves, but manning the till was stressful. None of the workplaces were able to hire her at the end of the internship, and the Public Employment Service couldn't find an internship that might lead to employment. Ida received activity compensation, and with it came a requirement to report back to the Public Employment Service lest she lose her benefits. All the energy she wanted to spend on looking for a job went into those never-ending reports and contacts with various people at the Public Employment Service and the Swedish Social Insurance Agency.

In the end, Ida had to sort out her own livelihood. One day, her husband saw a note at the grocery store about a cleaning job.

'I thought: I have to find the courage to apply. I've been going for several years to the Public Employment Service and got nowhere.'

She sent off an application to the cleaning agency, went in for an interview, and got to start right away. The job turned out to be cleaning the offices of the Public Employment Service. Ida returned to the same office where she had long been registered, but this time as an employee at a job she had found herself — without the help of the public employment officers.

'I just said, "hey there". They are really glad I'm working there, and happy with the cleaning. They say it's never been so clean before.'

If autists were in the majority, society would look different. In school, there would be fewer group projects, lower noise levels, smaller classes, greater predictability, and lower demands on flexibility. Workplaces wouldn't be organised as open-plan offices, and conferences wouldn't include so many team-building exercises.

Unemployment rates are higher among people with a neuropsychiatric diagnosis than the population at large. Among American autists with a university education, 85 per cent are unemployed. According to Autism-Europe, more than 75 per cent of people with autism in Europe don't have a job. There are no exact figures for Sweden, but the Autism and Asperger Association estimates that the unemployment rate is higher than 50 per cent. The risk of suicide is nine times higher among autists than the rest of the population. And 88 per cent of women with a neuropsychiatric diagnosis suffer or have suffered from mental illness, according to a report from the organisation Attention. A big Swedish study indicates that the average lifespan is 16 years shorter for people with autism.

Those who believe that neuropsychiatric diagnoses are imaginary conditions in self-absorbed present-day people fail to make the connection to the pervasive societal changes that have taken place over the past 30 years, in schools and at work. Public life as we know it has changed in that the amount of sensory stimulation — and especially the noise level — has increased dramatically.

Hypersensitivity to sensory input is likely the biggest obstacle for autists in the workplace. In many professions, sound and stress levels are high and show no signs of abating. More and more workplaces are arranged as open-plan offices, even though research has shown that almost everyone — not just autists — feels uncomfortable.

Today, you can't move through a shop or restaurant or cafe without being exposed to loud music. In playgrounds outside preschools, staff lug out loudspeakers and let the children play to the sound of Avicii. There is music playing at the swimming pool. On the bus, passengers are watching YouTube videos without headphones. At the library, visitors talk on the phone. The quiet spaces are gone. There are no doors to close upon oneself.

At my workplace, speakers were recently installed in the lifts, from which our radio broadcasts are now streaming without pause. Anyone wanting to get away from the noise has to take the stairs.

Another obstacle for autists on the job market is the inability to sugar-coat their statements. Truth-tellers and whistleblowers are rarely popular with the boss. Demands on employees being pleasantly flexible and adaptable have grown. In a time when everyone is thought of as replaceable, of course the boss is likely to get rid of someone calling her a 'fucking fake', no matter how hard they work.

According to annual reports from the Swedish Work Environment Authority, demands in the workplace have been on the rise since the early 1990s. A fast-paced job market dominated by the proliferation of the gig economy, zero-hour contracts, and rationalisations requires top-performing individuals. Most of all, it's no longer enough for you to have one or a couple of strong competencies; you have to be multi-talented. This includes expectations on social skills, dealing with meetings in big groups, and being able to handle administration and finance.

People with autism — to an even greater extent than others — need a stable workplace with predictable working conditions.

The philosophy professor Jonna Bornemark, who has a son with autism, thinks that our way of organising society has become inhuman. She considers the question of what kind of people we are expecting to build our society to be an urgent one.

Her book *The Renaissance of the Immeasurable* is a crusade against our time's fixation on measuring and documenting. That fixation has led our work to become a search for perfect processes that are fully repeatable and independent of who is involved. On business's dream job market today, anyone can swiftly be brought in and put to work without any learning curve whatsoever. All the manager has to do is give the employee the manual.

The rigid criteria that are used in the name of rational organisation assume that all employees are the same. And the more you assume that all people are the same — and thus interchangeable — the worse the conditions become for the autists, who are different from the majority. In the boxes provided, there is no space for the adjustments an autist needs, nor is there any way to take advantage of their strengths.

In school, there is room for adjustment for students with neuropsychiatric diagnoses, but that mainly applies to loud, extroverted boys with ADHD. The quiet autistic girl suffering from the high noise level doesn't get the same treatment. Parents of autistic girls who keep it together at school speak of difficulties simply getting school representatives to believe in the diagnosis. The teachers don't see the girls breaking down at home after the end of the school day.

A computer might be amazing at doing calculations, says Jonna

Bornemark, but it has no judgement. Yet the capacity for judgement exists in every human being. It's a hidden bank of knowledge that we have forgotten how to tap into. We have instead come to equate judgement with subjective opinion, which may vary from individual to individual. And yes, a subjectivity without shared morals can turn into scattered opinion, prejudice, and arbitrariness. But if we fail to nurture common agreement and commonsense judgement, we will be forced to reinvent the wheel over and over again, in each new piece of documentation consisting of data that's been collected and analysed. How is that efficient?

I see a paradox in our time. Our knowledge of neuropsychiatric diagnoses is growing, while the space for being different keeps shrinking. In the era of algorithms, we search more than ever for deviations from what is assumed to be normal. Examples can be found even at the grocery store. The algorithm designed to help the store ensure the integrity of the self-checkout system identifies the movement pattern of the person holding the scanner. Wandering around among the shelves in a confused pattern is registered as an issue, and a person who moves that way is more often subjected to spot checks to see whether the items have been paid for. What is normal and rational is to walk straight to the correct shelf — not doing so is an anomaly. When algorithms replace human judgement, there is no room for considering each individual situation on its own unique terms. The view of what is normal and what is aberrant eats its way into everything.

The space for difference has shrunk.

Year after year, student surveys conducted by the Swedish Schools Inspectorate show that around one in four students in the fourth grade lacks a peaceful study environment. More than half of respondents state that other students are disrupting the order in the classroom.

In other words, a quarter of Swedish students suffer from the elevated noise level in schools. The survey is conducted twice a year, and the results are consistent over time.

The Education Act stipulates that education should be designed in such a way that all students have a school environment that is safe and offers the peace and quiet required for study. Yet even though the problem is well known, the disruption continues. According to the Schools Inspectorate, there is no clear pattern in the types of schools or geographical areas that struggle with an unsettled study environment. Regardless of where students live or which school they go to, a quarter of them lack the peace and quiet required for study. There is no scientific evidence that these 25 per cent also have autistic traits or a sensitivity to sound, but it doesn't seem unlikely that this could be the case.

'It's highly individual,' says a teacher interviewed by the public broadcaster Sveriges Television in February 2020. Some students prefer complete quiet. Others work better with a bit of sound around them.

Though according to the survey report, all students prefer silence. I search for interviews with students who feel that their schoolwork benefits from loud sounds and talking, but I can't find any.

Personally, I didn't suffer from a high noise level in the classroom, as no one was allowed to speak during class in my school in the 1980s. Any student who disrupted the others' concentration was kicked out of the classroom. If a student continually disrupted the order in class, they were placed in a separate so-called 'observation class'. Schools are no longer allowed to do that.

Since I went to school, the prevailing pedagogy has been transformed from a model where teachers led the class from their desk at the front of the classroom, and students were expected to sit and listen quietly, to one where students are supposed to seek knowledge themselves, often in group projects. It's not uncommon for several different activities to be going on at the same time in the classroom and for the noise level to be high. A student who is bothered by their classmates' talking is told to wear hearing protection. Talking has become the norm, and the quarter of students who need silence are forced to adapt.

In the Facebook group for women with autism, I read about their alienation. Members write about longing for a job but not being able to get onto the job market. They can't find work because they can't take just any job. They share experiences and ask each other for advice. Working in a warehouse — has anyone tried that?

One group member started medical school. Becoming a doctor had been a long-held dream, and she was ecstatic at getting in, given that it required outstanding grades. But the course used a method known as 'inquiry-based learning', which required students to make a lot of choices on their own. They had to seek information, choose which books to read, and identify relevant content themselves. They worked in groups on case studies where they were assigned imaginary patients and had to figure out together what the patients suffered from.

The method worked for students who were social, extroverted, liked working in groups, and did well in a study environment without much of a framework. But it wasn't suitable for a person who needed clear boundaries. Unable to sort through the material, the member of the Facebook group explained, she was soon inundated. Having to identify relevant books and questions on her own required so much effort that she ran out of energy. By the time she was ready to sit down with the books and understand their content, there was none left. She dropped out and gave up on her dream of becoming a doctor.

In the group, grown, intelligent, eloquent people speak of not being able to find their place in the world. The demands for flexibility, social competence, and stress tolerance are too high. The slow, predictable jobs that would suit them don't exist.

I read about people struggling to elbow their way into a system that wasn't made for them. They are dependent on the goodwill of public institutions, but these institutions don't understand them.

Many are caught in a web of government agencies that take up all their time and energy. I see them forced to place their lives in the hands of employment officers, coaches, caseworkers, decision-makers, counsellors, support persons, and occupational therapists, who are often replaced and whom they each time have to convince that they need help all over again. I don't read a single testimony from anyone who has been helped by their contacts with the Social Insurance Agency and the Public Employment Service.

I wish I could tell them to rethink, to give up all these fruitless battles they cannot win, and attempt to disentangle themselves from the government agencies' web. I wish I could tell their parents to be more present in their lives and not leave them to their fate just because they are legal adults. The modern ideal where each individual alone is responsible for their home and livelihood doesn't work for someone who isn't given access to the job market. The message to people with autism is that they should live on benefits. At the same time, their applications are rejected.

The support system, as it is currently designed, is not adapted to an invisible disability. Yet nor is it reasonable to expect a society where all government-agency representatives have a strong grasp of a diagnosis that varies from individual to individual, may be partially masked, is difficult to detect, and expresses itself in many different ways. That's wishful thinking. The best thing for many autists would be to give up the fight against an unscalable bureaucracy and take help from their family and civil society instead. Living together across generational lines, helping each other financially. But modern society isn't built like that. People don't have enough money, and everyone is expected to take care of themselves.

In Sweden, an individual can break free from dependence on their family, private institutions, and charitable organisations. When the state takes responsibility, the individual is freer. But as support from family and civil society decreases, dependence on the state increases. And as our common welfare system is increasingly dismantled, it leaves a void. Help is nowhere to be found, neither from family and civil society nor from policymakers. What is someone supposed to do who can't break into the job market, is turned away by the public authorities, and receives no support from their parents?

Not until there is a proper improvement in the knowledge of autism and an increased awareness that not everyone functions the same way will there be adequate help for people with an autism diagnosis. I wish I could tell the members of the Facebook group not to wait for that societal transformation. There is no guarantee that it will come. Your lives are here and now.

An autist who follows society's rules for how a person with autism should act is forced to live out their life in phone queues while waiting for benefits and various forms of support that must be reapplied for on a regular basis and can be revoked at any moment. It's a life of phone calls, follow-ups, re-evaluations, rejections, appeals, savings, withdrawn support, new rules, new points of contact. That's no way to live. As far as possible, you have to take care of your own adjustments. As far as possible, you have to break free and create your own happiness. In light of the development thus far, it's hard to believe that the future will offer a more autism-friendly society, with a slower pace, smaller groups, reduced stress, and more-predictable jobs.

Sven Bölte conducts autism research and educates public-sector employees in neuropsychiatric diagnoses. Those who turn to his organisation KIND — the Center of Neurodevelopmental Disorders at the Karolinska Institute — are municipalities, administrative regions, or the national government when they need to raise the competency of, for instance, social workers and case officers at the Social Insurance Agency or the Public Employment Service.

We are sitting in KIND's offices on Gävlegatan in Stockholm, speaking about the future of young people with autism. Bölte shakes his head when the environment in schools comes up in conversation. The demands for personal responsibility and flexibility that are currently being put on schoolkids would never be accepted by the adults working in schools, he says. The union would step in.

Bölte is passionate about making the World Health Organization's classification framework ICF — the International Classification of Functioning, Disability, and Health — the standard across society. ICF is a refined diagnostic instrument, a tool for classifying functional capacity.

As an example, Bölte brings up the relatively large number of students who no longer go to school, so-called 'truants'. He would rather not use the term, because it stigmatises the student and implies a certain laziness. He prefers to say 'problematic school absences'. With ICF as a tool, it would be possible to investigate more precisely what's happening to the students in the school environment, what strengths and weaknesses they have, and why they aren't going.

School is an artificial environment in which society has decided that children should be able to function. It's loud, crowded, and unpredictable, and students with a neuropsychiatric diagnosis are often bullied. Refusing to go doesn't appear all that strange. Why would anyone want to be part of such a setting?

'For perhaps 10–15 per cent, it doesn't work at all. That's a lot, and that's the group we are talking about.'

Bölte thinks that schools should take as their starting point the lowest level of stimuli that students with a diagnosis can handle. But that's not currently the case. Instead, they use the average as a baseline and leave students to adjust. At the same time, schools for students with special needs are few and far between.

The general trend is that schools today place a greater responsibility on their students than in the past. They are expected to function at a high level and be entirely flexible. For children with autism, it's often very difficult to handle changing instructions and information at short notice.

'It starts with the schedule,' Bölte points out. 'Different times each day, in many different locations. New schedules are handed out all the time. Students are doing special assignments and group projects — schools are like little universities. Eleven-year-olds are expected to lead their own student–teacher conferences.'

He is happy about the progress being made, like the government deciding that all teachers must now undergo basic training in neuropsychiatric diagnoses. The decision came after KIND published a countrywide survey of the knowledge among school personnel that showed deplorable results.

With ICF as a tool, it would be possible to more precisely measure a student's strengths and weaknesses, and differentiate between what students really know and what they are able to show in school.

But sometimes Bölte doubts that training from organisations like KIND will have a broader impact on society. It takes years to truly learn to understand autism.

In countries like the US and the UK, understanding of autism is developing faster, he says. They are better at seeing strengths and turning the diagnosis into something positive. There are, for instance, companies and organisations — including recruitment and placement agencies as well as autism hiring programs — that specialise in the competencies of individuals on the spectrum, because they have understood that there is much creativity and reliability to be found there.

He is frustrated with the focus on diagnostic assessments in Swedish society and the lack of general knowledge. He says that older, well-read autists often know more than young psychologists at the clinics. Nor is there much help to be found once the assessment is done. Even though it would often be enough to make only small adjustments in day-to-day life, he says, taking Greta Thunberg as an example of an autist who flourished once she found her place. But there isn't enough interest in adapting to the individual. Often, not much happens. Bölte argues that autism is something that needs to be approached on a societal level — it can't be solved by the child and adolescent psychiatric services or adult rehabilitation alone.

To those who ask if there isn't a problem with overdiagnosis, he likes to say that we might eventually land on an accurate proportion of the population with neurodivergence of around 20 per cent. Then, more people will understand that this is a bigger challenge for society as a whole.

Bölte says that the way we treat people with autism and ADHD as well as their families reflects the degree of civilisation in society. An area where we have achieved a higher degree of civilisation, he says, is with LGBTQ issues. These have been given a lot of attention and priority in recent years; there has been a lot of training.

'If we were to get there with autism and ADHD as well, it would no longer be possible for someone to say that they don't know anything about it, or don't care. When it comes to LGBTQ issues, you can no longer say: "I don't know anything, we can't do anything about that, it doesn't exist, it's not my responsibility." But it's still possible to say that about neuropsychiatric diagnoses.'

Bölte is impatient but sees that things are moving in the right direction. Perhaps it will be another couple of generations before a real jump in knowledge has taken place.

As a researcher, he also works part-time at Curtin University in Perth, Australia. In Australia, there are solutions for school absences. Home-schooling is allowed. Parents can hire a private tutor, teach their child themselves, or make other arrangements. In Sweden, home-schooling is prohibited.

Bölte, who is Swedish but was born and raised in Germany, sees a strong tradition of conformist thinking in Sweden. There is a belief that both children and adults are all the same, an unwillingness to see differences between people. This doesn't lead to increased equality but has the opposite effect — as those who are different are made invisible and excluded.

But in people with a neuropsychiatric diagnosis, there might also be a tendency to become resigned to one's situation.

'Unfortunately, experience tells us that no prince is going to ride in and save you,' he says bluntly. 'Of course, you need to be able to make reasonable demands, but you can't expect society to change so much that you are saved. It'll never happen.'

By reasonable demands, he means having the same right to work as others and the same right to go to school with reasonable adjustments.

In Sweden, neuropsychiatric diagnoses still come with a certain stigma. It was only in 2021 that the rules changed to allow autistic individuals to enlist in the police or the armed forces. The former bans on applying to the police academy and doing military service existed even though many autists are dutiful, reliable, and obey rules to the letter — qualities that should be valuable to these organisations.

Individuals with autism must still submit a doctor's note on the 'current status' of their diagnosis when applying for a learner's permit.

THE PATRONESS OF IMPOSSIBLE CAUSES AND HOPELESS CIRCUMSTANCES

What distance must I maintain between myself and others if we are to together construct a sociability without alienation, a solitude without exile?

ROLAND BARTHES, *HOW TO LIVE TOGETHER*

The notion that a diagnosis can be a superpower has become a contemporary cliché, overused by those who want to counteract stigma. It's a nice thought, and I like my own strengths, but rarely do I feel like I have a superpower.

What's more, some of my strengths are entirely useless. I have the capacity to be harsh if I choose to, but this has mostly been a burden. Often, I haven't even realised that I'm being perceived as unforgiving.

Instead, I think I have just been clear, if perhaps expressing myself a little too forcefully in my eagerness to stress my point and make myself understood. But neurotypicals are so easily hurt.

When I learnt that people could take offence from the things I said, I tried to compensate with politeness and caution in order not to hurt anyone. I'm always unsettled by situations where other people are impolite — when someone isn't giving proper thanks, for instance. I apprehend a coming disaster.

In the world of neurotypicals, it's reasonable to lie, but getting angry is forbidden. Nothing scares them more than people losing it and raising their voice. Personally, I'm not afraid of openly unpleasant people. They are clear and comprehensible. Yet anger is just becoming more and more unfashionable. By that I mean the kind where people step into the world as themselves, unleashing a fit of rage face to face — not online hate speech behind the safety of a screen. Becoming furious is a sure way to be declared incompetent and shunned. The one who gets angry has always lost.

I remember fights I have had in my life, how they have ended with me huddled up, hiding my head under my arms. Unable to speak, all but unreachable.

At 42 years old, I find out that this is called a 'shutdown'. The inner pressure that builds from the stress of navigating a world difficult to comprehend may eventually cause a person to crack. The frustration and the feeling of being cornered are too strong, leading the person to shut down. The brain is overloaded and can no longer process what is happening. By contrast, a reaction to this overload directed outwards is called a 'meltdown'.

I remember the times I have been duped. I trusted too much in the words; it didn't even cross my mind that they could be untrue. I couldn't see that what the person said wasn't reflected in their face. So naive and gullible, the perfect victim. And yet I'm not. The details that didn't tally, the parts where the story didn't add up — those I noticed right away. And so I asked, over and over again.

§

The American author Patricia Highsmith had certain set ideas about what she liked. She enjoyed Bach's *St Matthew Passion*, worn-in clothing, running shoes, silence, Mexican food, fountain pens, Swiss Army knives, weekends without social obligations, Kafka, and being alone.

She didn't like the music of Sibelius, art by Fernand Léger, live concerts, four-course meals, TVs, the Begin–Sharon regime in Israel, loud people, people who borrow money, being recognised by strangers in the street, fascists, and thieves.

For a period as a young woman, Highsmith was anorexic. Her peers at university described her as hard to get to know, a private person with a strong sense of integrity. She had decided early on to become an author; writing was the only thing that eased her recurring nightmares. Later in life, she suffered bouts of depression. People who met her perceived her as shy and doggedly stubborn.

When her lesbian romance novel *The Price of Salt* was published in 1952, under the pseudonym Claire Morgan, the paperback cover featured the words 'explosive material' — a bait typical of the genre, meant to draw in a male audience. In the mid-1980s, the person behind the pseudonym was revealed to be one of the world's most skilful crime writers, famous for her books about the talented gentleman-psychopath Mr Tom Ripley.

The novel's story about the department-store assistant Therese, who falls in love with the refined housewife Carol, is at least partially based on true events. Highsmith did work in a department store for a time in order to pay for a course in psychoanalysis that she was taking in an attempt to make herself become heterosexual. One day, a poised blonde woman in a mink coat walked into the toy section to buy a doll. It was a brief encounter between a saleswoman and her customer, but in her diary Highsmith describes how, later that same night, in a feverish state, she scribbled down the basic plot of the novel in just an hour or two.

During the 1950s and 60s, Highsmith lived alone in Britain and France. Her books sold better in Europe than in the US. She stayed in France for 13 years, but never learnt to speak French. To her beloved Siamese cats, she spoke in a language of her own. She liked snails, often carrying around a great number of them, which she fed with lettuce. Visitors reacted to the food she served, which was barely edible, and her garden, neglected and overgrown. She never shook hands when saying hello. Eventually, she fled the French tax authorities and moved to Switzerland, where she lived out her days.

In all parts of life, not just love, Highsmith preferred women over men. Men who were annoyed by her described her as a man-hater, a particularly rude one who never missed a chance for a snide remark. Women described her differently.

In Andrew Wilson's biography *A Beautiful Shadow*, the therapist and author Vivien De Bernardi, a friend of Highsmith, says that the latter showed clear signs of autism. Highsmith couldn't go shopping in supermarkets, because the sensory stimuli overwhelmed her. The people were too many and the noises too loud. If someone moved an object in her home, she had to put it back in its rightful place immediately.

She had motor difficulties, could never find her way, was hypersensitive to sounds, struggled to communicate, and didn't understand nuances in social interactions.

De Bernardi describes her as a quiet person when it was just the two of them. If there were other people present, Highsmith behaved like a defiant child and could say the very first thing that popped into her head. She couldn't keep herself from speaking her mind; it was as though she lacked an inner control mechanism, and didn't understand when she hurt others' feelings.

§

'Doris just doesn't deal with human beings very well. She deals with cats very well.'

The words belong to an assistant to the author Doris Lessing, one of the literary greats of the 20th century, who as well as writing many novels also wrote several books about cats.

When people spoke of Lessing as an individual, they often used words like 'headstrong', 'difficult', and 'irreverent'. She was known as a lone wolf who abandoned her husband and children to live as a free intellectual on her own terms. Her radical, independent choices made her a feminist role model — yet she described herself as selfish and immoral, a bad citizen who wasn't suited for marriage.

After studying Lessing's biographies and authorship, the psychiatrist Michael Fitzgerald places her on the autism spectrum.

Rarely has a Nobel Prize–winner looked more annoyed than when a Reuters reporter stopped the almost-88-year-old Lessing in the street in October 2007 to tell her that she had been awarded the prize for literature.

'Oh, Christ,' she sighed, with a dismissive wave.

'But this is a recognition of your life's work,' the reporter tried.

'I've won all the prizes in Europe, every bloody one. I'm delighted to win them all, the whole lot ... It's a royal flush,' Lessing replied over her shoulder as she stepped through the gate to her home.

Later, when she found out that the Swedish Academy had called her the 'epicist of the female experience', she snorted: 'Ridiculous. But I guess they have to say something.'

My husband and I divorced, and it was both of our faults but mostly mine. I never overcame my anxiety, and assumed it had to do with our relationship. So I thought I might be happier with someone else.

I thought I was being authentic when I didn't put on a false front in his presence. But my honesty and failing capacity to imagine the world through his eyes kept me isolated from him. I lived encapsulated and powerless while he slipped further and further away.

I was autistic and didn't know it. I didn't understand that similarity isn't the same as intimacy. I didn't understand that a romantic relationship is also a performance. I could never restrain myself; I thought I could always live out my emotions in his company, regardless of their nature. The fact that he didn't do the same to me — that he didn't place all his darkness on my lap — I didn't notice.

One person can't constantly be burdening the other with their unfiltered anxiety and sorrow. No matter how bone-tired you are, sometimes you have to stick on a smile and keep your mouth shut. Put on a brave face and a bit of a show. Let the other person have their interests, instead of brooding over why they care about such trivial things and how that difference makes your union less complete. One must actively consider how the other person is feeling and doing. You don't need to talk about everything and always be digging into the pain.

We divorced, and I tattooed an image from a 15th-century fresco depicting the Catholic saint Rita of Cascia onto my forearm. St Rita is the patroness of impossible causes and hopeless circumstances — the only one left when God himself has given up. She is often depicted holding a skull, with roses and a stigmata on her forehead. After the death of both her husband and her two sons, she lived as a nun in an Augustinian convent. To this day, her incorrupt body lies preserved in a church in the Italian town of Cascia.

A while after my tattoo healed, I read that St Rita is also the patron saint of unhappy marriages. But by then it was too late.

I said a silent prayer. It was an incantation, a sentence stuck in my head, a string of words silently repeated with every step I took towards the bus stop after being discharged from a weekend at an inpatient psychiatric care facility:

I wanted so badly for you to like me.

They were the words of a child. A sentence so laughably simple and free from all suspense and finesse that I didn't want to repeat it to my therapist, in whom I had confided that it was looping through my mind. It popped up one day and took up space. Then it wouldn't go away. It repeated itself over and over in my brain, the only words I could think as I spent my weekend at the psych ward after the divorce.

I shared a room with a woman who had worked at a poetry festival and lay whimpering throughout the night. Personally, I refused to get out of bed. When I finally stepped out into the hallway, there was an old lady with a large wound on her head whom the staff were chasing back and forth. Everyone else stood watching with their backs pressed against the wall.

How dirty and miserable it was in the mental-health services in Sweden the welfare state. Even the magazines were tattered — damp, old, thumbed issues of some illustrated weekly.

I remember the doctor who said that on a suicidal-ideation scale from one to ten, I was a two — and I remember that a brief disappointment ran through me. He was right, but I wished he had assessed me as just a little more suicidal. Otherwise, what was I doing there?

'You shouldn't pretend to be fine in order to be let out sooner,' a mental-health nurse said in a Finland Swedish dialect as we exchanged a few words in the hallway, and I sensed a threat in his voice.

And then there was the mental-health nurse Zian, who may have saved me a little — the one who came to sit by my bed and tried to convince me to get up. I explained that my husband had been seeing someone else. (That I, too, had been unfaithful, I neglected to mention.) He replied that I was the prettiest girl in Stockholm, and so there was no reason to be sad. In the next breath, he took it back: he couldn't possibly know, he hadn't met all the girls in Stockholm. But he reckoned I might be one of the prettiest.

It was funny. I managed a smile.

Then he told me that he was in the same situation as me: his woman had cheated on him — 'can you believe how long she's been doing it?' — and he had exiled her to an air mattress on the floor, but they hadn't separated yet. We agreed that she could go to hell and that he was doing the right thing by waiting and seeing.

And I felt better after meeting Zian, better than after my medication — so much so that I could step out to eat the repulsive food served in the yellow room where everything smelled of ash and the cigarette lighters were chained to the walls. There was an old man, halfway turned into a corpse, slouched deeply over his soup, and out in the corridor was the lady with the big wound on her head who kept wanting to take her trousers off. And then there were the young girls with cuts all over their arms and black hair hanging lank and greasy under their hats. They flocked together outside the closed door to the staff room, waiting for someone to come out, and now the air trembled and thickened with anxiety and all this mingling madness, it became hard to breathe, and the walls crept closer.

There was a leader, of course, a woman who spoke incessantly with everyone. I was terrified of accidentally meeting her gaze, prompting her to go after me. She walked around raging at the Pride parade, saying it was unfair that the gays and the dykes had their own procession, that we should have one, too, a parade for mad folk — a parade for the mentally ill straight through town is what we should have.

It was like fiction, a long unreality, my weekend in inpatient care. And I don't know why I look back on it as a comedy, because I had fallen apart and was truly, acutely unhappy, so beaten down and annihilated that I couldn't get up.

We divorced and I spent long evenings on the couch in the living room playing Candy Crush the whole time so I wouldn't have to exist. The candy poured across the screen as papers were signed and furniture divided up, without me really being there. My friends asked why we were splitting up, and I couldn't answer because I didn't understand it myself. I said something about us becoming like siblings, but really it had always been that way — that's why we belonged together. All I knew was that we had begun to fight each other and couldn't stop.

My husband, who had always been annoyed at my piles of paper, now told me he would miss them.

I moved.

What if I had known how uniquely ill equipped I was for a life of constantly separating from the kids? What if I had known how it would feel to continue parenting together, after the person closest to me had assumed a new shape, transforming into a stranger with whom to negotiate logistics?

The worst part was how we tried so hard and for so long to stay together, and yet we failed. Others said it meant the divorce was true, because we had really tried. But I saw the futile struggle as a sign that we didn't actually want to part. It would have been easier to mourn a swift, rash mistake. Now I had to mourn that slow, dumb, desperate trying, too. All that time, all our willingness and inability.

On the days when I regret the divorce the most, I imagine that I'm paying for the mistake with my autistic loyalty. Other people move on and build new lives. I don't. I stay.

The wrong choices I have made remain, like blocks of stone in the road.

Those who seek out the clinic in Hagsätra almost always have a history of anxiety and depression, my psychologist tells me. These are known as secondary symptoms. You can become depressed from being autistic. If you don't interpret reality like others around you, there is a significantly greater risk that you will feel unwell. For many, the depression eases once they are diagnosed because they have finally found the source of their darkness.

Anxiety is the human feeling of not being in true harmony with oneself, says Søren Kierkegaard. He has plenty more thoughts on the essence of anxiety, but this one stays with me. Such has been my life. Something is wrong, something ain't right. Masking it bores a hole in one's soul. That's really what Kierkegaard is saying.

The experience of being a stranger to oneself is absurd, Kierkegaard writes in his book *The Concept of Anxiety*. Perhaps it is particularly absurd to an autist without any knowledge that she is different.

Often, autistic adults who undergo their assessment late in life have already tried a number of treatments without success. Neither medication nor cognitive behavioural therapy nor psychoanalysis is going to help an autistic person who doesn't know about their autism.

Around the same time as the field of child psychiatry began to take an interest in neurology, the view on anxiety and depression in adults underwent a similar change. In the West, we started teaching that depression was caused by an imbalance in the brain, which could be remedied with medication. There was talk of 'clinical' or 'chronic' depression, a congenital and unchanging condition. The *reasons* why people were depressed, which had previously been sought through conversations with psychoanalysts, became less important. With the new pills, the patient's childhood could be disregarded.

At the same moment that antidepressants had their big breakthrough, solution-oriented cognitive behavioural therapy (CBT) became increasingly common. In Swedish and British public healthcare, CBT is now the predominant form of therapy. Through exercises aiming to change behaviours and disrupt thought patterns, CBT treats the symptoms of depression. But like pharmaceuticals, it does nothing to address the roots of the condition.

Sigmund Freud said that neurotic symptoms have a meaning that is related to the life of the people who produce them. It sounds self-evident, but in the prevailing view of mental illness in our time there is an idea that it simply comes over us, like catching a cold. Personally, I didn't 'have' depression; I felt anxious about experiencing the world differently, functioning differently, and not understanding myself.

The individual's story about their life problems that they outline on the psychoanalytic couch is unique. It reflects their place in the world and their relationship to themselves and others. Medications and CBT erase the human subject, as the same methods are assumed to work for everyone.

The aim of psychoanalysis isn't adaptation but to achieve liberation — one's unique individuality as a human being, the psychoanalyst Anna Krantz explains in an article in the newspaper *Dagens Nyheter* in February 2020. And liberating one's person — that is, finding one's own unique individuality — is no doubt a more appealing prospect than ridding oneself of depression through medication or exercises. But an autistic person who isn't aware of their condition will reach no insight through either psychoanalysis or CBT.

In order to speak freely and associatively in the company of a psychoanalyst, you must know what you are feeling. An autist doesn't. The difficulty in making sense of one's feelings is part of the diagnosis. The degree of unawareness is too high for the autist to be able to cure herself by merely opening her mouth and beginning to speak in another's company. Am I afraid, empty, downcast, irritated? No idea.

Nor does CBT fully work even if the autist knows her diagnosis. Autism doesn't go away with exercises or thinking. Trying to overcome the difficulties by subjecting oneself to them has a very limited effect. You can practise looking other people in the eye when speaking to them, but it will always require the same effort. And no one rids themselves of their hypersensitivity to loud sounds by spending time in noisy environments.

EPILOGUE

And hear us, world, that likes and condemns, so quick to throw flowers or stones. We have never sought what you praise, nor shunned what you are used to loathing.

ERIK AXEL KARLFELDT

The psychologist in Hagsätra walks me out into the waiting room. The diagnostic assessment is complete. He wishes me good luck and hands over a written summary.

I walk underneath the concrete canopies in downtown Hagsätra back to the metro, passing the grocery store, the sculpture *Girl with a Ball* by its empty pond, and the pastry shop. And this time I find the way. I finished. I solved the mystery.

On the metro ride home, I watch a TikTok video by the young autistic artist Nicole Parish. She paints insects and runs the account @soundoftheforest, calling herself a mysterious tree nymph. In the clip, she sits deeply absorbed, wearing large noise-cancelling headphones, painting a butterfly. Light floods into her studio from a nearby window. The butterfly is incredibly rich in detail. With her left hand, she traces thin, almost imperceptible lines with the brush. Her right hand moves like that of a conductor; she shakes it and splays her fingers wide, controlling the rhythm of the work with her stimming. She is deeply immersed and completely free. I have never seen a happier image of an autistic woman, and the clip makes me cry all the way to Gullmarsplan. Imagine if my youth could have been like that.

What remains for me now? Unmasking.

I watch Greta Thunberg stim dancing in the documentary *I Am Greta* and think about the ballerinas and how dancing and stimming are the same language.

I close my eyes and rewind my own tape again, seeing the clues from my childhood and teenage years and life as a young adult. They line up, one by one. What if I had known sooner? How would my life have turned out? I tell myself that the thought is impossible — during my childhood, there was no such thing as a girl with high-functioning autism. No one could have given me a diagnosis. My life thus far is not a series of years lost. But still. The signs were there. I mourn not being able to decipher them before. Instead, I repressed everything that was true in me and kept striving towards further defeat. If I had known, many mistakes could have been avoided. There would have been fewer blocks of stone in the road.

Having grown up with undiagnosed autism is to have suffered difficulties that didn't exist. Female high-functioning autists, as a recognised category, didn't exist. And yet I was one of them.

I remember a sentence from a children's book — one of those ugly, pedagogical books from the '70s, illustrated with thick black lines. It was about deafblind people. 'Being able to neither see nor hear is to live in a world of silence and darkness,' it said. I could both see and hear but often felt as though I lived in that world.

My diagnosis is the best thing that has happened for my self-esteem. It became a wave that carried me onwards. After those three months in

Hagsätra, I went from failed neurotypical to regular autist. The joy and relief in finally fitting in was indescribable. I understood who I was and could accept it and find peace. Only once I received my diagnosis did I feel certain that I was in fact a real human being.

After the elation of that initial period, I noticed something had happened inside me. A calmness slowly crept up on me, a long exhalation that I could feel in my body and hear in my own voice. I spoke more slowly and with more confidence. My anxiety went down and I lowered the dosage of my antidepressants.

Perhaps it wasn't just the diagnosis but also my age, but I started to cultivate and like my own quirky sides. I found the strength to say no to things I had previously thought I must do. The mere idea that I would never have to go skiing again made me so happy that I kept thinking it, over and over. I realised that I don't have to bear everything. I found the courage to ask for help and explain to old men in bike shops that what seems easy-peasy in their eyes is not so for everyone and that I cannot pump a tyre myself. I ate chicken korma for dinner every day for a week without scruple. I watched the same Marx Brothers film nine times over simply because I wanted to. I began to ignore the way non-autists mistake autistic behaviour for arrogance and kept my headphones on when inside. I realised that therapy is meaningless unless the therapist knows autism. I shrunk my life, peeling away things and musts, protecting everything that made me feel good. I became proud of my difference.

Even so, after my diagnosis I found myself in an interstice. I could see my difficulties and how they had affected me throughout my life. I realised that I had spent 42 years adapting and trying to function in a way that didn't really work for me. The problems that remain are that I'm very capable in certain areas, which constantly obscures my difficulties, and that I have spent a lifetime practising adaptation.

In this interstice, I continue to behave in the ways I have learnt. I mimic and conform. Out of old habit and ingrained experience, I continue to mask and make an effort in social situations, at the expense of my own energy. I work full-time, am a single mother every other week, and am always on the brink of exhaustion. When I tell others that I'm autistic, I'm met with indulgent smiles or a comment on how it seems everyone has a diagnosis these days.

It's hard to settle into my new role when there is so little knowledge about autistic adults. I don't have the energy to educate people all the time. I want to live a free, authentic, autistic life without having to defend myself.

A few times, I seek help from an occupational therapist. She visits me in my home, and we talk about how I can save energy in order to have enough to both work full-time and be a parent. She is kind and accommodating, and I get some general advice. But we don't connect.

After our sessions are over, she calls me for a follow-up. She doesn't say it, but I can hear that she is interviewing me off a questionnaire. How well do I feel that the objectives for our sessions have been fulfilled? I try to help her with an answer, picking a number between one and ten. I gather that this is a form of documentation that her employer requires of her, an evaluation that will be stored somewhere and used later on as the basis for some statistic. Everything is and must be measurable.

I'm the exception; I know that now. It's my brain that works differently compared to others'. I'm the one who deviates from the norm. Nevertheless, I think everyone should be like me. It's the others who are wrong, and I'm right. You are the ones who are weird, while I'm normal. You have an impaired ability to interact socially with me, not the other way around.

To me, people who are not autists can appear cowardly, dishonest, and scared of conflict. They never say what they think; instead, they imply and act all evasive until the conversation turns murky and tangled. They have low moral standards for themselves and others, rarely practise what they preach, and aren't even ashamed of it. They gossip behind their friends' backs and are obsessed with what others think of them. They deny the truth. They break promises. They say one thing and do another. Why are they rushing all the time, and why can they never give a straight answer to a simple question?

I know that as an adult you are expected to accept that the people around you tell white lies, maintain a facade, and don't always mean what they say. It's normal to presume that other people might not be fully authentic. But I struggle with it. How do they justify their inconsistency when searching their own conscience? Do they ever?

I have spent my life pretending, playing the neurotypical game, and figuring out social codes. I'm fed up with it. I wish the autist's way could be the norm. I wish that all this pretence wasn't normalised.

Who is the regular human being to whom the norm refers? Who is the 'normal' — the one for whom the rational models are built?

Neurotypical individuals make up the norm because there are more of them. Autists are a minority and as such we are forced to adjust to the reality around us. For many, it's a lifelong struggle.

But deficits and disabilities only exist in relation to an environment where some other way of functioning has been chosen as the yardstick. An autistic person — or one with any form of otherness — only becomes an anomaly when she tries to fit in. Beyond any and all contexts, she is complete in herself.

I return to Simone Weil. She writes that the most important and overlooked spiritual need of humanity is to take root. A human being has roots when she has a 'real, active, and natural participation in the life of a community which preserves in living shape certain particular treasures of the past and certain particular expectations for the future'.

Each person needs many roots, Weil writes. 'It is necessary for [her] to draw well-nigh the whole of [her] moral, intellectual, and spiritual life by way of the environment of which [she] forms a natural part.'

It's a new year. One day when parents are invited to join the children in class, I visit my daughter's school. I sit on the classroom couch and watch as the children colour in drawings of animals. When the bell rings for lunch, we walk to the canteen where chilli fish and boiled potatoes are on the menu. We choose the table farthest into the corner. Sitting there, alone, is a girl in another class. I sit down across from her. On her plate are three pancakes. No toppings. She looks at me.

'I get to eat this because I have autism,' she says, and puts a piece of pancake into her mouth.

'Me, too,' I say.

ACKNOWLEDGEMENTS

I would like to thank my original publishers Lawen Mohtadi and Richard Herold for their tireless encouragement and deep commitment to the text.

Thank you to Tove Larsmo for invaluable editorship and to Fanny Frost for sharp-eyed proofreading.

Thank you to the groups Psykjuntan and Svarta Cirkeln for support, fellowship, and homework.

Thank you to Kristin Lundell and Caroline Hainer for beauty, cookies, and a bit of gambling.

Thank you to Negar Josephi, Alex Haridi, Carina Berg, Åsa Wallinder, Johan Korssell, Malin Wallebom, Linda Leopold, Nina Bennet Crafoord, and Peter and Joel Bernhard.

Thank you to Ann-Louise and to Barbro, who said: 'Dare to trust in your longing.'

Thank you to the San Michele Foundation for the space and the view.

Thank you to the Facebook group.

Thank you to everyone who allowed me to interview them.

To autistic women everywhere: live long and prosper.

BIBLIOGRAPHY

INTRODUCTION

Sylvia Plath. *The Bell Jar*. New York: Harper & Row, 1971.

THE AUTISTS

Love on the Spectrum, season 1 episode 4. Directed by Cian O'Clery. Northern Pictures, 2019.

Kristiina Tammimies and Anna Hellquist. 'Genetisk variation och genetisk testning vid autismspektrumtillstånd' (Genetic Variation and Genetic Testing in Autism Spectrum Disorder). KIND — the Center of Neurodevelopmental Disorders at the Karolinska Institute, 18 March 2021. <https://ki.se/media/169824/download>

Katarina A. Sörngård. *Autismhandboken* (The Autism Handbook). Stockholm: Natur & Kultur, 2018.

Oliver Sacks. *An Anthropologist on Mars: seven paradoxical tales*. New York: Vintage Books, 1995.

Jenny Widell and Eva Klint Langland. 'Förlorade år — rapport från byråkratins väntrum' (Years Lost: a report from the waiting rooms of bureaucracy). Autism and Asperger Association in Sweden, 2021. <https://www.autism.se/media/i1qeoka3/forlorade_ar_webb.pdf>

THE INVISIBLES

Svenny Kopp. Interviews with the author. 17 March and 22 October 2020.

Sarah Britz. 'Vidkärrs barnhem värst i landet' (Vidkärr Orphanage Worst in the Country). *Göteborgs-Posten*, 23 December 2012. <https://www.gp.se/nyheter/göteborg/vidkärrs-barnhem-värst-i-landet-1.681795>

Magnus Berg. *Ett ömmande hjärta: Vidkärrs barnhem i Göteborg 1935–1976 och därefter* (An Aching Heart: Vidkärr Orphanage in Gothenburg, 1935–1976 and after). Gothenburg, Sweden: A-Script Förlag, 2014.

Svenny Kopp and Christopher Gillberg. 'Vem söker barnpsykiatrisk öppenvård? Fem års nybesök vid en barn- och ungdomspsykiatrisk mottagning i Göteborg' (Who Seeks Child Psychiatric Outpatient Care?: first visits during five years at a child and adolescent psychiatric clinic in Gothenburg). *Läkartidningen*, vol. 96, no. 46, 1999: p. 46. <https://lakartidningen.se/wp-content/uploads/OldPdfFiles/1999/20237.pdf>

Svenny Kopp and Christopher Gillberg. 'Girls with Social Deficits and Learning Problems: autism, atypical Asperger syndrome, or a variant of these conditions'. *European Child & Adolescent Psychiatry*, vol. 1, no. 2, 1992: pp. 89–99. <https://pubmed.ncbi.nlm.nih.gov/29871391/>

Kaja Nordengen. *Your Superstar Brain: unlocking the secrets of the human mind.* London: Piatkus, 2018.

Alison Lurie. *Clever Gretchen and Other Forgotten Folktales*. Lincoln,
NE: iUniverse Inc., 2005.

HOLY FOOLS AND REFRIGERATOR MOTHERS

The Queen's Gambit, season 1 episode 3, 'Doubled Pawns'. Directed by
Scott Frank. Flitcraft Ltd, Wonderful Films, and Netflix, 2020.
Julia V. Douthwaite. *The Wild Girl, Natural Man, and the Monster:
dangerous experiments in the Age of Enlightenment*. Chicago:
University of Chicago Press, 2002.
Roy Grinker. *Unstrange Minds: remapping the world of autism*. New
York: Basic Books, 2007.
Natalia Challis and Horace W. Dewey. 'The Blessed Fools
of Old Russia'. *Jahrbücher für Geschichte Osteuropas*,
vol. 22, no. 1, 1974: pp. 1–11. <https://www.jstor.org/
stable/41044822?searchText=blessed+fools+of+old+russia>
Christine Trevett. 'Asperger's Syndrome and the Holy
Fool: the case of Brother Juniper'. *Journal of
Religion, Disability & Health*, vol. 13, no. 2, 2009:
pp. 129–50. <https://www.tandfonline.com/doi/
abs/10.1080/15228960802581537?journalCode=wrdh20>
Marlies Janz. *Elfriede Jelinek*. Stuttgart, Germany: Sammlung Metzler,
1995. Cited in Leland de la Durantaye. 'On Cynicism, Dogs, Hair,
Elfriede Jelinek, and the Nobel Prize'. *Harvard Review*, no. 29, 2005:
pp. 146–53. <https://www.jstor.org/stable/27569096?search
Text=On+Cynicism,+Dogs,+Hair,+Elfriede+Jelinek+
and+the+Nobel+Prize>
Edith Sheffer. *Asperger's Children: the origins of autism in Nazi Vienna*.
New York: W.W. Norton & Co., 2018.
Herwig Czech. 'Hans Asperger, National Socialism, and "Race
Hygiene" in Nazi-era Vienna'. *Molecular Autism*, no. 9, 2018:

pp. 1–43. <https://molecularautism.biomedcentral.com/
articles/10.1186/s13229-018-0208-6>

Temple Grandin and Richard Panek. *The Autistic Brain: exploring the strength of a different kind of mind*. London: Rider Books, 2013.

Irina Manouilenko. Interview with the author. 27 April 2020.

Lina Zeldovich. 'How History Forgot the Woman Who Defined Autism'. *Spectrum News*, 7 November 2018. <https://www. spectrumnews.org/features/deep-dive/history-forgot-woman-defined-autism/>

Irina Manouilenko and Susanne Bejerot. 'Sukhareva — Prior to Asperger and Kanner'. *Nordic Journal of Psychiatry*, vol. 69, no. 6, 2015: pp. 479–82. <https://pubmed.ncbi.nlm.nih. gov/25826582/>

Irina Manouilenko. 'Autismspektrumtillstånd hos vuxna — biologiska aspekter' (Autism Spectrum Disorder in Adults: biological aspects). The Karolinska Institute, 2013. <https://openarchive. ki.se/xmlui/handle/10616/41605>

'Medicine: The Child Is Father'. *Time*, 25 July 1960. <https://content. time.com/time/subscriber/article/0,33009,826528-1,00.html>

LOST IN THOUGHT

Simone Weil. *Gravity and Grace*. Translated by Emma Crawford and Mario von der Ruhr. London: Routledge Classics, 2002.

Kristofer Ahlström. 'Varför blir män besatta så fort de ska göra något?' (Why Are Men So Obsessed as Soon as They Are Doing Domething?). *Dagens Nyheter*, 9 February 2020. <https://www. dn.se/kultur-noje/varfor-blir-man-besatta-sa-fort-de-ska-gora-nagot/>

Lars-Olof Strömberg. 'Märta, 12, har rummet fullt med käpphästar' (Märta, 12, Has a Room Full of Hobbyhorses). *Expressen*, 9

February 2020. <https://www.expressen.se/kvallsposten/marta-
12-har-rummet-fullt-med-kapphastar/>

Carolina Alexandrou. Interview with the author. 4 March 2020.

Linn Sundberg. Interview with the author. 10 March 2020.

Ebbe Schön. *Troll och människa: gammal svensk folktro* ('Trolls and
Men: old Swedish folklore). Stockholm: Hjalmarson & Högberg,
2008.

Selma Lagerlöf. 'Bortbytingen' (The Changeling). In *Troll och
människor* (Trolls and People). Stockholm: Albert Bonniers
Förlag, 1915.

Michael Fried. *Absorption and Theatricality: painting and beholder in
the age of Diderot*. Chicago: University of Chicago Press, 1980.

Michael Fitzgerald. 'Beatrix Potter Was on the Spectrum'. *ResearchGate*
(preprint), March 2021. <https://www.researchgate.net/
publication/349733806_Beatrix_Potter_was_on_the_
spectrum>

Michael Fitzgerald. *Autism and Creativity: is there a link between
autism in men and exceptional ability?* London: Routledge, 2004.

AN ATTACK ON ALL SENSES

Katarina Frostenson and Aris Fioretos. *Skallarna* (The Skulls).
Stockholm: Bonnier Essä, 2001: p. 43.

Virginia Woolf. *Mrs Dalloway*. London: Vintage Classics, 2016.

Stuart Murray. *Representing Autism: culture, narrative, fascination*.
Liverpool: Liverpool University Press, 2008.

Gunilla Gerland. *En riktig människa* (A Real Person). Lund, Sweden:
Studentlitteratur, 2010.

Lina Liman. *Konsten att fejka arabiska: en berättelse om autism* (The
Art of Faking Arabic: a story about autism). Stockholm: Albert
Bonniers Förlag, 2017.

Beata Ernman, Malena Ernman, Greta Thunberg, and Svante
  Thunberg. *Our House Is on Fire: scenes of a family and a planet in
  crisis.* London: Penguin Books, 2020.
Temple Grandin. *Thinking in Pictures.* New York: Doubleday, 1995.
Frida Anter. 'Ätstörningar kopplas till autismspektrumtillstånd' (Eating
  Disorders Connected to Autism Spectrum Disorder). *Special
  Nest,* 20 February 2017. <https://www.specialnest.se/forskning/
  atstorningar-kopplas-till-autismspektrumtillstand>

THE AUTOMATONS

Simone Weil. *Gravity and Grace.* Translated by Emma Crawford and
  Mario von der Ruhr. London: Routledge Classics, 2002.
Katarina Wikars. *Det som gick mig ur händer* (That Which Got Out
  of My Hands), 10 February 2011. Radio Sweden P1, 2011.
  <https://sverigesradio.se/artikel/4340705>
Viktor Shklovsky. 'Art as Device'. Translated by Alexandra Berlina.
  Poetics Today, vol. 36, no. 3, 2015: pp. 151–74. <https://read.
  dukeupress.edu/poetics-today/article-abstract/36/3/151/21143/
  Art-as-Device>
Ida Hallin Mellwing. Interviews with the author. 24 March 2020 and
  11 April 2021.
Sigmund Freud. 'The Uncanny'. In *The Uncanny.* Translated by David
  McLintock. London: Penguin Books, 2003.
John Ajvide Lindqvist. *Let the Old Dreams Die.* Translated by Ebba
  Segerberg. New York: Thomas Dunne Books, 2013.
Mara Lee. *När Andra skriver — Skrivande som motstånd, ansvar och
  tid* (The Writing of Others: writing conceived as resistance,
  responsibility, and time). Gothenburg, Sweden: Glänta
  Produktion, 2014.

THE UNBEARABLE WEIGHT OF BEING

Svenny Kopp. Interview with the author. 17 March 2020.

TOO MUCH FAITH IN WORDS

I Am Greta. Directed by Nathan Grossman. B-Reel Films, 2020.
'Greta Thunberg: inspiring others to take a stand against climate
    change'. *The Daily Show with Trevor Noah*. Comedy
    Central, 11 September 2019. <https://www.youtube.com/
    watch?v=rhQVustYV24&t=118s>
C.L. Lynch. 'Caring for Your NT During Social Isolation'.
    NeuroClastic, 2 April 2020. <https://neuroclastic.com/caring-
    for-your-nt-during-social-isolation/>
Lars Melin. *Polletten som trillade ner: metaforer: hur förstår vi dem?*
    (The Penny That Dropped: metaphors — how do we make sense
    of them?). Stockholm: Norstedts, 2012.
Julie Brown. *Writers on the Spectrum: how autism and Asperger
    syndrome have influenced literary writing*. London: Jessica
    Kingsley Publishers, 2010.
Jac den Houting. 'Why Everything You Know About Autism
    Is Wrong'. TEDxMacquarieUniversity, 1 November 2019.
    <https://www.youtube.com/watch?v=A1AUdaH-EPM>

THE AUTISTIC BRAIN

A Quiet Passion. Directed by Terence Davies. Hurricane Films and
    Potemkino, 2016.
Temple Grandin and Richard Panek. *The Autistic Brain: exploring the
    strength of a different kind of mind*. London: Rider Books, 2013.

Temple Grandin. *Thinking in Pictures*. New York: Doubleday, 1995.

Kristiina Tammimies and Anna Hellquist. 'Genetisk variation och genetisk testning vid autismspektrumtillstånd' (Genetic Variation and Genetic Testing in Autism Spectrum Disorder). KIND — the Center of Neurodevelopmental Disorders at the Karolinska Institute, 18 March 2021. <https://ki.se/media/169824/download>

Sven Bölte. Interview with the author. 9 September 2020.

Frithiof Dahlby. *Helgondagar* (Saints' Days). Stockholm: Diakonistyrelsens Bokförlag, 1958.

Frithiof Dahlby. *De heliga tecknens hemlighet: om symboler och attribut* (The Secret of the Holy Signs: symbols and attributes). Stockholm: Verbum, 1999.

Søren Kierkegaard. *The Concept of Anxiety: a simple psychologically oriented deliberation in view of the dogmatic problem of hereditary sin*. Translated by Alastair Hannay. New York: Liveright Publishing, 2015.

PEER PRESSURE

Erik Axel Karlfeldt. 'Löskekarlarnes sång' (The Song of the Vagabond). In *Fridolins lustgård och Dalmålningar på rim* (Fridolin's Garden and Dalecarlia Paintings in Verse). Stockholm: Wahlström & Widstrand, 1901: p. 91.

Alex & Sigges Podcast, episode 406, 'Anti-Greta', 28 February 2020. <https://podtail.com/en/podcast/alex-och-sigges-podcast/406-anti-greta/>

Lucy Diavolo. 'Greta Thunberg Wants You — Yes, You — to Join the Climate Strike'. *Teen Vogue*, 16 September 2019. <https://www.teenvogue.com/story/greta-thunberg-climate-strike-teen-vogue-special-issue-cover>

Lisbet Palmgren. *Diktarnas, barnens och dårarnas språk* (The Language of Poets, Children, and Fools). Stockholm: Natur & Kultur, 1997.

Jonna Bornemark. *Det omätbaras renässans — En uppgörelse med pedanternas världsherravälde* (The Renaissance of the Immeasurable: facing up to the world domination of the pedants). Stockholm: Volante, 2018.

Hélène Cixous. *Three Steps on the Ladder of Writing*. Translated by Sarah Cornell and Susan Sellers. New York: Columbia University Press, 1993.

Katarina Frostenson. *K*. Stockholm: Polaris, 2019.

Simone Weil. 'Human Personality'. In *Simone Weil: an anthology*. Translated by Richard Rees. London: Penguin Classics, 2005.

Simone Weil. *The Need for Roots*. Translated by Arthur Wills. London: Routledge Classics, 2001.

Michael Fitzgerald. *The Genesis of Artistic Creativity: Asperger's syndrome and the arts*. London: Jessica Kingsley Publishers, 2005.

Rosemary Dinnage. *Alone! Alone!: lives of some outsider women*. New York: New York Review Books, 2004.

Francine du Plessix Gray. *Simone Weil*. London: Weidenfeld and Nicolson, 2001.

Ioan James. *Asperger's Syndrome and High Achievement: some very remarkable people*. London: Jessica Kingsley, 2006.

John Cody. *After Great Pain: the inner life of Emily Dickinson*. Cambridge, MA: Harvard University Press, 1971.

I LOCK MY DOOR UPON MYSELF

Gunilla Gerland. *Autism — relationer och sexualitet* (Autism: relationships and sexuality). Lund, Sweden: Studentlitteratur, 2011: p. 39.

Joyce Carol Oates. *I Lock My Door Upon Myself.* New York: Ecco Press, 1990.

Christina Rossetti. 'Who Shall Deliver Me?'. *The Complete Poems.* Penguin Classics, 2001.

Damian Milton. 'On the Ontological Status of Autism: the "double empathy problem"'. *Disability and Society*, vol. 27, No. 6, 2012: pp. 883–7. <https://www.tandfonline.com/doi/abs/10.1080/09687599.2012.710008>

Catherine J. Crompton et al. 'Autistic Peer-to-Peer Information Transfer Is Highly Effective'. *Autism*, vol. 24, No. 7, 2020: pp. 1,704–12. <https://journals.sagepub.com/doi/full/10.1177/1362361320919286>

E.T.A. Hoffmann. 'The Sandman'. In *Tales of Hoffmann*. Translated by R.J. Hollingdale. London: Penguin Books, 1982.

Jutta Emma Fortin. *Method in Madness: control mechanisms in the French fantastic*. Amsterdam: Rodopi, 2005.

INSULA

Lewis Carroll. *Alice's Adventures in Wonderland* and *Through the Looking-Glass, and What Alice Found There*. London: Penguin Books, 1998.

Joanne Limburg. *The Autistic Alice*. Newcastle upon Tyne, Britain: Bloodaxe Books, 2017.

Julie Brown. *Writers on the Spectrum: how autism and Asperger syndrome have influenced literary writing*. London: Jessica Kingsley Publishers, 2010.

SCHOOL AND WORK

Björn Afzelius. 'Balladen om K' (The Ballad About K). Track 4 on *Bakom kulisserna* (Behind the Scenes). Nacksving, 1979. <https://www.youtube.com/watch?v=sK9GnJYSBvI>

Din hjärna (Your Brain), season 1 episode 5, 'Lika men unika' (Similar but Unique). Directed by Niklas Nyberg. ITV Studios Sweden, 2019.

'Se mig, förstå mig, ta mig på allvar — En undersökning om situationen för flickor och kvinnor med neuropsykiatriska funktionsnedsättningar (NPF) och psykisk ohälsa' (See Me, Understand Me, Take Me Seriously: a study of the situation for girls and women with neuropsychiatric disabilities and mental illness). *Riksförbundet Attention*, 9 September 2020. <https://issuu.com/familjelyftet/docs/rapport_-_flickor-kvinnor-npf_och_psykisk_oha_lsa_>

Tatja Hirvikoski, Sven Bölte et al. 'Premature Mortality in Autism Spectrum Disorder'. *British Journal of Psychiatry*, vol. 208, no. 3, 2016: pp. 232–8. <https://pubmed.ncbi.nlm.nih.gov/26541693/>

Jenny Widell and Eva Klint Langland. 'Förlorade år — rapport från byråkratins väntrum' (Years Lost: a report from the waiting rooms of bureaucracy). Autism and Asperger Association in Sweden, 2021. <https://www.autism.se/media/i1qeoka3/forlorade_ar_webb.pdf>

Lotta Olin. 'En fjärdedel av femteklassarna saknar studiero' (One-in-Four Fifth-Graders Lack the Peace and Quiet to Study). *SVT Nyheter*, 28 February 2020. <https://www.svt.se/nyheter/lokalt/dalarna/en-fjardedel-av-femteklassarna-saknar-studiero>

Jennifer Alm. 'Blekingelärarna om studiero — finns hörselkåpor och skärmskydd i klassrummet' (Teachers in Blekinge on a Peaceful Study Environment: there are hearing protection and screen

protectors in the classrooms). *SVT Nyheter*, 28 February 2020.
<https://www.svt.se/nyheter/lokalt/blekinge/lararen-jenny-om-studiero-valdigt-individuellt>
Sven Bölte. Interview with the author. 9 September 2020.

THE PATRONESS OF IMPOSSIBLE CAUSES AND HOPELESS CIRCUMSTANCES

Roland Barthes. *How to Live Together*. Translated by Kate Briggs. New York: Columbia University Press, 2012.
Andrew Wilson. *Beautiful Shadow: a life of Patricia Highsmith*. London: Bloomsbury, 2003.
Patricia Highsmith. *The Price of Salt*. New York: W.W. Norton & Co., 2017.
Michael Fitzgerald. 'Doris Lessing Was on the Spectrum'. *ResearchGate* (preprint), March 2021. <https://www.researchgate.net/publication/349693966_Doris_Lessing_was_on_the_spectrum>
'British Author Doris Lessing Reacts to Nobel Win'. Reuters, 13 October 2007. <https://www.youtube.com/watch?v=vuBODHFBZ8k>
Kajsa Haidl. 'Psykoanalysen är tillbaka — nu längtar allt fler unga efter divanen' (Pyschoanalysis Is Back: more and more young long for the couch). *Dagens Nyheter*. 2 February 2020. <https://www.dn.se/kultur-noje/psykoanalysen-ar-tillbaka-nu-langtar-allt-fler-unga-efter-divanen/>
Johan Eriksson. 'Psykoanalysen är absolut ett alternativ till kbt' (Psychoanalysis Is Definitely an Alternative to CBT). *Dagens Nyheter*, 6 February 2020. <https://www.dn.se/kultur-noje/johan-eriksson-psykoanlysen-ar-absolut-ett-alternativ-till-kbt/>

Cecilia Jacobsson. 'Skarp och obruten' (Sharp and Unbroken). *Dagens Nyheter*, 8 February 2008. <https://www.dn.se/arkiv/kultur/skarp-och-obruten/?site=desktop>

EPILOGUE

Erik Axel Karlfeldt. 'Löskekarlarnes sång' (The Song of the Vagabond). In *Fridolins lustgård och Dalmålningar på rim* (Fridolin's Garden and Dalecarlia Paintings in Verse). Stockholm: Wahlström & Widstrand, 1901: p. 91.